Turn Off the

Hunger Switch

Naturally

Paul Rivas, M.D.

with

E. A. Tremblay

A CONCISE EDITION OF

TURN OFF THE HUNGER SWITCH

AVERY · A MEMBER OF PENGUIN PUTNAM INC. · NEW YORK

Turn Off the Hunger Switch Naturally

The Revolutionary New Program

That Resets Your Brain Chemistry

for Real Weight Loss

Without Cravings or Hunger

Most Avery books are available at special quantity discounts for bulk purchase for sales promotions, premiums, fund-raising, and educational needs. Special books or book excerpts also can be created to fit specific needs. For details, write Putnam Special Markets, 375 Hudson Street, New York, NY 10014.

a member of
Penguin Putnam Inc.
375 Hudson Street
New York, NY 10014
www.penguinputnam.com

Library of Congress Cataloging-in-Publication Data

Rivas, Paul.
Turn off the hunger switch naturally / Paul Rivas with E. A. Tremblay
p.   cm.
"Previously published as Turn off the hunger switch"—T.p. verso.
Includes bibliographical references and index.
ISBN 1-58333-154-9
1. Weight loss.   2. Appetite.   I. Tremblay, E. A.   II. Rivas, Paul.
Turn off the hunger switch.   III. Title.
RM222.2.R553   2003   2002034291
613.7—dc21

Printed in the United States of America
1   3   5   7   9   10   8   6   4   2

BOOK DESIGN BY MEIGHAN CAVANAUGH

Contents

Turn Off the Hunger Switch Naturally

Introduction

I am a bariatrician, a doctor who treats people who find it difficult to control their weight. And today I am a *successful* bariatrician. My patients actually lose weight and keep it off. But it hasn't always been so.

Like most weight-loss doctors, when I first began my practice, I immediately ran up against a brick wall. I had gone through standard medical training at a good medical school, so I offered everyone who came to see me the standard medical advice I had learned: Eat less and exercise more. The problem was that my advice didn't work. Most of my patients weren't getting any thinner, and those who were didn't stay that way for long.

Then one patient, Roy M., came in one day and did something that would forever change the way I practiced medicine.

Roy had been coming to my office for years, desperately looking for a way to control his weight, but he just couldn't seem to make any progress. The problem was that he loved Italian food, craved it so much, in fact, that he felt completely helpless to resist when in the presence of a beckoning bowl of pasta. Finally, at my wit's end, I accused him of being a bad patient. He didn't bother to point out my failure as a doctor. He simply asked me for pills to control his appetite.

If you have ever gone to your family physician, or even a bariatrician, and asked for diet pills, you already know this story. Pills are precisely what you do not get. What you probably do get is a stern look (or, if you're lucky, a fatherly one) and a pamphlet that tells you to count your calories, cut down your fat intake, and exercise more. What you probably also get is the feeling that your doctor does not take your problem seriously. You are not like his other patients, patients who are genuinely sick.

And so it was with Roy. I told him that I did not believe in diet pills and had never suggested them in ten years of practice.

Why not?

Until recently, most diet pills were prescription medications that came from the amphetamine family. These drugs are powerful appetite inhibitors, but they are also dangerous and addicting. People who use them over an extended period of time often become restless and nervous. Many develop the "shakes," a chronic and noticeable trembling of the hands. Insomnia is common. Overdoses can cause depression, psychosis, and death. These were not drugs I would give to people I care about. And I care very much about my patients. I didn't realize at the time that science was already discovering new tools—many of them natural supplements as powerful as medications—to fight obesity.

As for Roy, I was convinced that, for some odd reason, he was choosing ravioli over self-esteem and good health. Losing weight, I thought, was simply a matter of making better choices and keeping one's self under better control. Not such a difficult thing for a person to do. After all, I controlled my eating habits, didn't I? Surely his temptations were no worse than mine.

Or were they?

Finally frustrated and out of patience, Roy handed me a copy of a report by Dr. Michael Weintraub. That moment was the beginning of a long evolution in my thinking that has changed Roy's life, the lives of my patients, and, perhaps most of all, my own.

In my years of practice since then, I've treated nearly 12,000 patients for their overweight condition, with close to a 95 percent success rate. All of those patients have driven home for me one fact that may contradict everything you have ever heard on the subject: Dieting and exercise have nothing to do with weight loss.

I know it sounds unlikely. I know it goes against common sense. But it's true. Don't take my word for it. Just look at the world around you.

Diet books are perennial best-sellers, even though they very often contradict one another. One proposes high carbohydrates, another high proteins, still another high fats. Some claim that simply balancing your meals will do the trick. Others suggest changing your eating habits according to your blood type or the season of the year. In the meantime, we spend millions of dollars on treadmills, tummy-toning exercise machines, and health club memberships.

Unfortunately, despite all this effort, we don't seem to be losing any weight. Nearly everyone who loses weight through diet and exercise gains it back within five years.

In my own practice, patients often come to me in utter confusion and despair after years of exhausting exercise and restricted eating with little or no weight loss to show for it. In fact, many have watched in horror as the needle on the scale actually moved *upward* when they cut their calories back. They feel weak and out of control.

"What's wrong with me?" they'll say. "What diet should I be on and how much should I exercise?" Or: "Maybe I should just give up and accept myself as I am."

My answer is usually not what they expected to hear. In fact, it's something that most people have never heard before: The size of your meals doesn't matter, but the size of your appetite does. It's not the degree to which you consume food, but the degree to which you crave and desire food that controls your weight. It's not so much the steaks, chocolate, and fries but rather the obsession with them that ultimately add fat to your frame.

Why? Insatiable hunger tells your body to go into its fat-storing mode. Your system feels the symptoms of starvation, so it stops "wasting" precious calories by burning them and stockpiles them instead.

So, I tell them, "Don't worry about eating that piece of chocolate but rather how much you crave it."

And what controls how much you crave and obsess over food? It has nothing to do with your diet; it has everything to do with your parents. It's not your exercise program that matters; it's your genetic program. The solution to your problem doesn't lie in willpower, self-control, or pushing away from the table. It lies in turning off your appetite, and your appetite center is located in your brain.

Once you do that, chocolate and sweets will instantly lose their appeal. You'll feel full after eating only a small portion of a meal. Food thoughts and compulsive eating stop. It's instant, dramatic, and works exceptionally well.

So put away your weight-loss books, throw away your tummy toners, and learn how to turn off your hunger switch. The day of the diet is over.

1

Hard Facts About Soft Tissue

Fat is unhealthy.

You already know this. You see it on television; hear it on the radio; read it in books, magazines, and newspapers. Every lethal disease you can think of seems to have some connection with eating red meat, dairy products, sauces, and pastries. Responsible health organizations the world over recommend a diet high in fruits, grains, and vegetables, and low in beef, milk, butter, and eggs.

The warning is clear: Putting too much fat into your stomach will make you sick—but so will putting too much fat *around* your stomach.

How much is too much? When we glance in the mirror,

Are You in the Danger Zone?

If you're carrying excess pounds, your health is in serious jeopardy. Too much fat *can* kill you.

How much is too much?

Until recently, doctors made that determination by looking at your body weight. Now there is a much more powerful tool for recognizing obesity. It's called the *body mass index,* or BMI. To determine your BMI, you have to do a little arithmetic. Take your weight in pounds and multiply it by 705. Divide that number by your height in inches. Then divide your answer by your height in inches again.

Weight × 705 ÷ Height in inches ÷ Height in inches = BMI

You can use this chart for quick reference:

BMI						
	HEIGHT					
WEIGHT	5'0"	5'3"	5'6"	5'9"	6'0"	6'3"
140 lbs.	27	25	23	21	19	18
150 lbs.	29	27	24	22	20	19
160 lbs.	31	28	26	24	22	20
170 lbs.	33	30	28	25	23	21
180 lbs.	35	32	29	27	25	23
190 lbs.	37	34	31	28	26	24
200 lbs.	39	36	32	30	27	25
210 lbs.	41	37	34	31	29	26
220 lbs.	43	39	36	33	30	28
230 lbs.	45	41	37	34	31	29
240 lbs.	47	43	39	36	33	30
250 lbs.	49	44	40	37	34	31

If your BMI falls within the range of 25 to 27, you're moderately overweight. From 27 to 30, you're obese. And if your BMI is over 30, you're seriously obese.

most of us don't see a problem. We may be sporting "love handles" or even a little "midlife paunch," but that, we tell ourselves, doesn't make us dangerously heavy. Obese people are more like those fat ladies in the circus. They look like Mama Cass Elliot or John Candy. *Those* are the people who die from being overweight.

Bariatricians will tell you otherwise. They've seen the numbers. They know that many people who call themselves "pleasingly plump" or "a little overweight" can fall well within the danger zone of obesity. And that is a very dangerous place indeed.

The Price to Your Health

If *you* fall within that zone, you are at greater risk for diabetes, heart disease, blood vessel disease, gall bladder disease, arthritis, and high blood pressure. You're also more likely to get cancer of the colon.

If you're an overweight male, your chances of developing prostate cancer are higher. If you're a plus-size female, you need to be more concerned about cancers of the ovaries and uterus than thin women do.

There is one glimmer of good news for overweight women: You're less at risk for heart disease than are your male counterparts—as long as you bear most of your extra weight below your waist, rather than around it. But your risk for breast cancer rises to one and a half times the average.

The picture becomes even more complicated—and frightening—if you're obese and pregnant. Your odds for bearing a baby with a debilitating birth defect double if you're seriously overweight (BMI of 27 to 30) and quadruple if you're danger-ously obese (BMI over 30). The two most common of these defects are spina bifida, which can paralyze a child, and anen-cephaly, a condition in which most of the brain is missing.

For some reason researchers don't yet understand, folic acid supplements reduce the risk of these defects in child-bearing women of normal weight but have no effect whatso-ever when taken by overweight mothers-to-be.

The Social Cost

Statistics concerning your health become worse and worse as your weight goes up, but health isn't the only issue. People who are noticeably overweight also have to contend with prej-udice, rejection, and scorn.

It's sad but true: If you suspect you were passed over for a promotion, denied a job, or simply not invited to a party be-cause of your size, you're probably right.

According to studies, a majority of college students claim they would rather marry a drug dealer or a thief than an obese person. Six-year-old children commonly call fat kids "dirty," "cheats," "liars," "ugly," and "stupid." And most surprising of all, even doctors often describe overweight patients as "weak-willed, ugly, and awkward."

So what are you supposed to do about all this? Some people simply decide to be proud of who they are, no matter how heavy they may be. They make a conscious decision not to lose weight. That's praiseworthy to a point. But it addresses only the issue of self-esteem, not health. And whatever you've heard in the news about being overweight *and* physically fit, exercise will improve only your circulatory and heart health. Your risk for cancer, diabetes, and arthritis remain dangerously high.

For most us, there can be only one decision: to take control of our lives and our health by losing weight.

Simple.

Simple? Are You Out of Your Mind?

"If losing weight is so simple, why does every approach I try work wonderfully for about five minutes before I start putting the pounds back on again?"

Good question. In fact, chances are good that there's not a weight loss plan or product on the market you haven't tested on yourself with lousy results. You've been through the struggle of trying to resist overwhelming cravings. You've starved yourself week after week, only to end up on the food binge of all food binges. You've forced yourself to jog, stair-climb, and aerobicize until you have the stamina of a cross-country runner. And you've swallowed enough "fat burners" to melt all the candles in the Vatican.

Worst of all, after turning your life into a boot camp and finally losing some weight, you've watched in horror as those lost pounds reappeared out of nowhere and attached themselves again, like stalkers waiting in ambush.

Now, you hardly put a crumb to your mouth, let alone overeat, yet you seem to get bigger and bigger. Imagining an entire lifetime on this merry-go-round is depressing to say the least.

To make matters even worse, we see people all around us who seem to maintain a healthy weight and slender body with no effort whatsoever. They're the same people who criticize us for not controlling our calorie intake. They eat what they want, when they want, and in whatever amount they want, but they never gain a pound. They look like a bunch of long-distance runners, though we know for a fact that many of them are couch potatoes. Exercise doesn't seem to make any difference.

What's going on here? Is there some fundamental, underlying physical difference between thin people and fat people? Science tells us there is.

Chips Off the Old Block

In 1988, the *New England Journal of Medicine* published the results of a Danish study of 540 people who had been adopted during infancy. The subjects of the study were divided into four groups: thin, normal weight, overweight, and obese. Their weights were then compared with those of their adopted parents and their biological parents. You might expect that the adoptees would mostly end up in the same weight class as that of their adoptive parents. After all, people in the same home would eat the same foods at the same mealtimes, and probably in similar quantities. The results, however, pointed in the other direction. Adoptees had a much stronger tendency to end up in the weight class of their biological parents.

Other research has yielded similar results. A 1986 study published in the *Journal of the American Medical Association* compared the weights of both adult identical twins and non-identical twins. If genetics was the important factor in body mass, then identical twins should grow up to be in the same weight class. And that's exactly what happened. The authors, using three different methods of analyzing their data, came to the conclusion that ". . . human fatness is under strong genetic control."

More recently, researchers have learned some of the ways in which genetics exert that control. At the University of California, scientists have discovered a gene that determines whether the fat you consume will burn off as harmless body heat or go into storage as adipose. In Britain, another team of investigators has found a protein, GLP-1, that signals the brain when you've had enough to eat. Similarly, a hormone, leptin, may be at least partially responsible for maintaining body weight at an unmoving level.

One of the most interesting and peculiar effects of genetics on body weight is a strong inherited tendency to like or dislike certain foods. Scientists announced this finding a few years ago at a meeting of the American Association for the Advancement of Science. Apparently, people divide broadly into three groups: supertasters, tasters, and nontasters. Because they've inherited more taste buds, supertasters actually taste more of the bitterness and sweetness in what they eat than do others. Nontasters can put virtually anything in their mouths to little or no effect. Naturally, the amounts and kinds of foods each group tends to consume are vastly different.

Heredity is so firmly connected to the problem of being overweight that 80 percent of the offspring of two overweight parents will become obese, as compared with only 14 percent of two parents who are of normal weight. But if heredity is so

The Role of Metabolism

"My metabolism is slow." Doctors hear it all the time from overweight patients. "If I eat any less, I'll die of starvation, but I still can't seem to lose a pound." This is usually the point at which the doctor's eyes will glaze over. He may be nodding his head in sympathy, but he's actually thinking, *She's deluding herself and making excuses. The less you eat, the more weight you lose. If you're not losing, then you're eating too much. End of story.* Meanwhile, she's thinking, *My body just doesn't burn calories the way other people's do. If I'm fat, it's because I have a built-in handicap.*

Who's right? Probably neither. When a person has a low metabolic rate relative to her size, studies show that she's also more likely to be carrying around too much body weight. The Pima Indians, who have, on average, slower metabolisms than nearly any other group of people in the world, also have the highest prevalence of obesity. But there is no clear evidence that a slow metabolism and obesity are related by cause and effect, only that the two conditions occur in the same people. There is much stronger evidence that they're both effects of a more fundamental cause: a genetic predisposition.

important, why do Japanese people still living in Japan generally remain thin, while their counterparts who have moved to the West become as fat as Europeans and Americans?

Heredity may create strong tendencies, but environment creates opportunities. Who knows how many Heifitzes and Perlmans lived and died before the invention of the violin? No matter how great the talent, if there is no fiddle, there is no fiddler. Likewise with obesity. In cultures where high-calorie foods are hard to come by, such as Japan and China, potentially overweight people remain thin. In the West, however, there is ample opportunity to eat fats, sugars, and starches, and we take advantage of it.

Situation Hopeful

Luckily for us, science is not all grim news. Bad genes don't make obesity inevitable, and we're beginning to understand the mechanism by which they do their dirty work.

If you give it some thought, you can probably pinpoint the specific time in your life when you began gaining weight. Perhaps it happened after some particularly stressful event, such as taking a new medicine and/or hormonal therapy; going through surgery, pregnancy, or a divorce; or suffering the loss of a loved one through death. Or it could have occurred simply as a result of reaching a certain age. You may have gotten heavy when you were young, or you may have been thin for the first several decades of your life before your weight suddenly spiraled out of control—despite the lack of any significant change in exercise or eating habits. As many overweight people say, it's as if a fat-storing switch had been turned on inside your body.

What a frustrating experience, to see your weight climbing and climbing, to find yourself obsessing over food all day every day, and to feel so completely powerless to stop the process! Yet it was exactly this situation that gave us the clues we needed to solve the mystery of obesity and the answers we needed to bring you the most life-altering news you'll ever hear:

There is a "fat-storing switch" in the body that can suddenly, and without warning, flip to the "on" position. But if you know how, *you can just as suddenly turn it off again!*

2

Hunting the Elusive
Fat-Storing Switch

n order to flip the switch, you first have to know where to find it, and therein lies the problem. For a very long time, we've been looking in all the wrong places.

The first place we tried was that hard-to-pin-down aspect of the human personality we call "character." We didn't look very closely at the conclusions we leapt to because we believed they were self-evident. Here was the logic: Whenever you eat, any energy you don't immediately burn you store as fat. The more you eat, the more you put into storage, and the fatter you become. Since many people manage to control their eating habits and remain at a healthy weight, people who don't obviously lack self-control. In other words, they have a *character flaw*.

The problem with this reasoning is obvious: Many, if not most, overweight people have spent much of their lives depriving themselves of food—often surviving on a ridiculously low intake of calories—despite experiencing very poor results in keeping the pounds off. What could show more self-discipline? And they bring this same determination to exercise. When it comes to strength of character, many thin people could take a lesson from their heavier brothers and sisters.

Next Stop, the Mind

All right, then, if the problem wasn't a character flaw, then perhaps it was subtler in nature. If the typical overweight person often deprived herself of food, it was still true that her behavior—frequently bingeing or chronically overeating—seemed to bring about her weight woes. So what was causing the behavior, some *psychological* problem?

When doctors tell their patients that losing weight is primarily a psychological problem, what are they really saying?

The theory goes something like this: Eating too much is a nervous response, a way to distract yourself from feeling uncomfortable. Any discomfort, including stress, depression, fatigue, anxiety, premenstrual syndrome, shyness, force of habit, or a hundred other situations, can trigger a food binge. So if you want to stop yourself from overeating, you simply need to find other ways of dealing with your discomfort. Bite your nails, blow your top, take up a hobby, or jog a few miles. But whatever else you do, learn to keep your mouth shut in the presence of food.

In other words, it was the same old "character flaw" argument, dressed up in slightly fancier clothing.

Could 12-Step Programs Be the Answer?

If the problem wasn't one of character, or one of mind, then perhaps we were looking in the wrong direction. Maybe the problem was actually one of *food*.

This reasoning led us to some pretty odd suspicions, the first of which was that food might be an addictive substance for some people. Some researchers even cited evidence for "withdrawal symptoms," the discomfort a food addict might experience if she didn't consume her addicting substance.

The addiction theory was a step up from the old way of thinking about obesity, in that it no longer victimized the victim, that is, it no longer pointed an accusing finger at overweight people to blame them for their problem. But on closer inspection, it didn't make much sense.

Any addicting substance hooks its prey by means of some chemical property in the substance itself. Alcohol, tobacco, and cocaine all produce biochemical changes in the human body that, among other symptoms, cause the body to need more of the addicting substance just to keep performing normal activities. With many drugs, a sense of euphoria reinforces the addiction. If you don't take the substance, you can't function, but if you do take the substance, you feel absolutely wonderful! The addiction turns insidious. The more you take, the more you need. This is called *tolerance*.

Food presents a different picture. We all need it to survive, but no one needs it more than anyone else. There is nothing in the food itself that addicts people to it. It doesn't produce real euphoria, and reports of "withdrawal symptoms" are at best questionable.

As for increased tolerance, if obese people were truly addicted, we would see them eating bigger and bigger meals day by day. Study after study shows that this just doesn't happen.

Not Addiction, but Obsession

Here is where the story gets interesting. Overweight people may not eat more food, but they sure do think more about it! Most are constantly preoccupied with the subject, even right after eating a large meal. They know their stomachs are full, but somehow they don't feel satisfied.

They think about food when they wake up in the morning, they think about it all through the day, and they think about it when they go to bed in the evening. Sometimes they even wake up in the middle of the night thinking about it! They crave, they binge, they pick, they nibble. And it's true: They sometimes eat when they're bored, anxious, stressed, irritable, or angry. But they also eat when they're relaxed and feeling good.

This is a portrait of neither a weak-willed person nor a typical addict. It is, however, very much like a picture of another class of patients: people with obsessive-compulsive disorder, or OCD. We've all heard about this disease. It leads to irrational, even ritualistic patterns of behavior over which the victim seems to have no control. An obsession with cleanliness that leads to compulsive hand washing is typical: People will wash their hands to the point of scrubbing off layers of skin, even though they know that what they're doing makes no sense and that it's hurting them. They just can't help themselves.

The similarity between OCD and food obsession suggested that we look for the hunger switch in another location altogether: the chemistry of the brain.

People with OCD have an underlying biochemical abnormality that may involve the brain substance *serotonin*. While we are not yet completely sure that a lack of sufficient serotonin in the brain lies at the bottom of this problem, we do know that selective serotonin reuptake inhibitors, such as Prozac™, Paxil™, and Zoloft™, help these patients enormously. Not only do patients stop their irrational behavior, but they stop obsessing as well.

Could obesity be treated in a similar way?

Ground Zero: The Hunger Switch

Appetite and weight control begin in a sort of control center of the brain called the *hypothalamus*. One of the "switch-

A Direct Approach: Brain Surgery

It's an old, accepted piece of wisdom that, when solving patients' medical problems, internists like to give medicine and surgeons like to operate. It should come as no surprise, then, that a new way to flip the hunger switch was presented at the Forty-ninth Annual Meeting of the Congress of Neurological Surgeons: brain surgery. David A. Vincent, M.D., presented his experimental findings after using a "gamma" knife (a machine that focuses several beams of gamma radiation on one point in the brain without opening up the skull) to irradiate the hypothalamus of thirty-six subjects. Follow-up observations ran for thirty-four weeks. The results of the experiment demonstrated that the weight thermostats of the subjects had been lowered to a healthy level, they all lost weight, and there were no adverse side effects. Only one problem: The subjects, in this case, were lab rats.

No, we're not quite ready to perform brain surgery as a weight-loss remedy for humans yet. But the study clearly demonstrated one thing: There *is* a thermostat in the brain that can turn off the hunger switch. It was great news for everyone concerned with helping people to lose weight. Fortunately, irradiating the brain is not the only option.

boards" in the center, known as the *ventromedial region,* is in charge of telling you when you've had enough to eat, that is, it's the place that sends you the signal that you're full. If this part of the brain is somehow badly damaged, enormous hunger and obesity always result. A laboratory rat will actually eat itself to death when its ventromedial region is destroyed.

The feeling of hunger comes from yet another control center, the *lateral hypothalamus*. If this area is damaged, loss of appetite and extreme thinness result.

By increasing brain levels of certain substances (including serotonin) that act as triggers for these two controllers in the hypothalamus, not only can we suppress appetite and overeating, but we can also liberate people from obsessing over food as well!

Suppose, however, that you don't really obsess over food. You don't spend all your time thinking about it, but now and again, maybe late at night, just before bed, you have a tremendous craving for something sugary or full of fat. It's interesting that the brain doesn't target vegetables or whole-grain foods when it springs one of these compulsions on you. It goes right for the unhealthiest thing on the menu, and perhaps with good reason.

Dr. Richard Wurtman, director of the Clinical Research Center at MIT, contends that the brain is actually medicating itself: "We observe that a sizable portion of obese subjects seeking assistance in weight reduction consume as much as half of their total daily intake as carbohydrate-rich snacks, and that the behavior is often associated with strong feelings of carbohydrate cravings. Conceivably, this appetite disorder reflects an abnormality in the process that couples carbohydrate consumption to the release of brain serotonin. Many patients describe themselves as feeling anxious, tense, or depressed before consuming the carbohydrate snack and peaceful or relaxed afterward. . . . Perhaps the subjects snacking on carbohydrate are unknowingly self-medicating."

In other words, they're trying to flip that switch.

From Bad Genes to Plus Size

Since the tendency toward being overweight is clearly inherited, it's a good bet that these "bad genes" do most of their dirty work by causing imbalances in brain chemistry. In turn, these imbalances cause excessive hunger or the inability to get full, cravings for salty or sweet foods, and compulsive eating even when you're not hungry.

But the story doesn't end there. When any of these symptoms appear, the brain signals the body to go into a starvation-storage mode. That means you become extremely efficient at using energy, leaving you able to store, as fat, almost everything you eat, and unable to break down any fat you've stored previously.

The Gene with a Double Whammy

It's bad enough that a gene could predispose us toward obesity, but it turns out that one such "fat" gene, called HMG I-C, is even worse: It also predisposes us toward cancer.

According to a laboratory study published in the May 2000 issue of *The Journal of Biological Chemistry*, that HMG I-C gene may cause benign tumors, called *lipomas*, to grow in fat tissue. In themselves, these tumors are harmless, but as they grow, many turn into a type of cancer called *malignant liposarcoma*.

The good news is that these tumors grow only in fat tissue—so now we have one more reason to keep body fat to a minimum.

That's why so many overweight people complain that they're eating like birds and still not losing weight. It also explains why a thin person, whose brain chemicals are in balance and whose internal engine burns fat faster than a race car burns gasoline, can eat whatever she wants and remain thin.

The mechanism works like a thermostat. When your genetic blueprint tilts your brain chemistry out of balance, the "fat-storing thermostat" in the hypothalamus rises to a high setting, and your body will do whatever it takes to reach the weight that setting demands. As you reach the setting, weight gain stops; people do not gain indefinitely. They hover within a couple of pounds around the set point.

If all this is true, then why aren't fat people born fat? How is it they can often pinpoint the time in their life when they gained much of their weight? Although imbalances in brain chemistry may be genetically determined, it often takes a trigger to set them off. These include stressful life events, like those mentioned in the last chapter. Unfortunately, simply getting rid of the trigger does not reverse the process.

We finally found the switch, nestled deep in the human brain. Now we had to figure out a way to turn it off.

3

From Switch to Switchboard

Back in the early 1990s, we thought we'd found the answer in a combination of two new appetite suppressants, phentermine and fenfluramine.

Phentermine is part of a drug family known as the *central adrenergics*. Phentermine increases the amount of two substances, norepinephrine and dopamine, in the brain. These, in turn, suppress appetite.

Fenfluramine causes cells to release another neurotransmitter, serotonin, directly into the brain, which also suppresses appetite. But serotonin performs a couple of other neat tricks as well: It lifts your mood, and it gets rid of cravings, especially for carbohydrates.

The Numbers Looked Good

How did we know all this? And how did we know that the drugs would actually work the way they were supposed to and help people to lose weight?

Preliminary studies had already been done on the medications in the late 1970s. Then, in 1989, the results of the first major study appeared in a highly respected British medical journal, *The Lancet*.

Research scientists had conducted a one-year-long experiment using the drug dexfenfluramine (a close relative of fenfluramine) along with a calorie-restricted diet on 822 overweight patients living all over Europe. The researchers wanted to know if obesity, which they called a "chronic, harmful disorder," could be safely treated with drugs on a long-term basis. After all, they reasoned, you could control chronic diabetes, high blood pressure, and high triglycerides with medication, so why not one of the chief underlying causes of these conditions?

The results were promising. At the end of the study, the European patients had enjoyed significant weight loss—more than 10 percent of their starting weight—with only minor, transient side effects.

Then, in 1992, Dr. Michael Weintraub and a team of scientists at the University of Rochester concluded a four-year study of phentermine and fenfluramine. Used together in low doses, the drugs helped over a hundred patients lose an average of almost 16 percent of their body weight in about eight months (as against a 4.6 percent average weight loss in a control group). That meant that a 200-pound patient taking these medications would have lost about 32 pounds!

The Snack Effect

Most overweight people actually eat about the same number of calories per day as their normal-weight counterparts, but they consume far more of those calories as starchy or sweet snacks. Why? Carbohydrates alter your mood by raising the level of serotonin in the brain. When that happens, all your worries seem to fly away. Medicines and supplements that raise serotonin do the same thing—without the added calories.

Dr. Judith Wurtman of the Department of Nutrition at MIT dramatically demonstrated this effect in a field study. She divided her subjects into two groups. People in the first group were given fenfluramine. Those in the second, the control group, were given placebos. The placebo takers ate, on average, five to six snacks per day. Patients using the medication, however, reduced their snack intake by 41 percent, without reducing their consumption of healthy foods at all. In other words, fenfluramine had selectively eliminated their desire to snack! Fortunately, there are combinations of natural supplements that do the same job, and you don't need a prescription to get them.

The following year, one of the world's most respected obesity researchers, Dr. Richard Atkinson, at the University of Wisconsin, reported the results of a study he had made. Atkinson had been giving phentermine and fenfluramine to a group of patients consisting of 57 men and 506 women and presented his findings at the annual meeting of the North American Association for the Study of Obesity. The Associ-

ated Press picked up the story. After three months, his patients had lost an average of 22 pounds. After six months, the
average jumped to 29 pounds, and after nine months, 37
pounds!

The News Gets Better

Weight loss was only part of the story. In forty-nine of the patients in Atkinson's study, blood pressure dropped to normal,
while twenty-four patients saw their cholesterol levels plum-
met. There was even some evidence that blood sugar had nor-
malized in several diabetic patients. "Dramatic stuff!" was the
way Atkinson put it in an article in the *Baltimore Sun* in 1993.

In 1994, a workshop conducted at the National Institutes
of Health concluded that ". . . pharmacologic agents may be
effective in reducing body weight over an extended period of
time," and that ". . . the drugs are effective and have a role in
the treatment of obesity."

The "Harvard Heart Letter" cited a study in which phentermine and fenfluramine were combined with diet counsel-
ing and behavior modification. The patients averaged 200
pounds at the start of the study and lost, on average, over 30
pounds.

The Big Letdown

We fell in love with these drugs, and who can blame us? We
even came up with a pet name for them: Phen-Fen. They
were available, by prescription, through drugstores, weight-

loss centers, the mail, and the Internet. Phen-Fen weight-loss programs were advertised on television, the radio, and in newspapers. I used the drugs extensively in my own medical weight-loss practice.

But the news wasn't all good. We knew from the beginning that Phen-Fen had side effects. Every medication does. A very small number of people in clinical trials, especially those taking higher doses, had complained of headaches, depression, sedation, excitation or insomnia, loose stools or constipation, blood pressure elevation, dizziness, dry mouth, and a mild difficulty with concentration or memory that seemed to come and go.

By far the most serious potential side effect of these drugs then known, however, was PPH, or primary pulmonary hypertension. PPH is an elevation of blood pressure in the vessels that go from the heart to the lungs. It's a serious, often fatal condition that affects about one in a million people in the general population, usually women in their mid-thirties. The use of these two drugs raises that number.

Three to four people out of every one hundred thousand who took these medications would contract the illness. About half of those would be reversible. In the remaining half, the patients would require heart-lung transplants to survive.

At first glance, these were frightening statistics, but not nearly as frightening as the fact that over 300,000 people in the United States were dying each year from diseases associated with obesity. Other common drugs had worse side effects that occurred more frequently. The benefits, we felt, were worth the risk.

All that changed, however, when we saw the results of

some small studies suggesting that fenfluramine and its close relative dexfenfluramine caused a side effect we had been completely unaware of: valvular heart disease. One group of researchers reported that as many as 30 percent of all those who had used the drugs developed some thickening of the valve that controls blood flow through the aorta, the heart's main blood vessel. This, obviously, could pose a grave danger to the health of these people.

The companies that manufactured the two drugs, commercially named Pondimin™ and Redux™, voluntarily recalled the products and immediately stopped producing them. Phentermine, commercially known as Ionamin™, never came into question. It is a very safe drug that is still in use today.

Since that initial research, no study has been able to duplicate the 30 percent figure, and many other studies have shown no significant rise in valvular disease with the use of these drugs. In my own practice, I saw neither PPH nor valvular disease in any of my patients—probably because I prescribed the drugs at only one-fourth the recommended dosage (with great results). Still, we won't know for certain about safety until larger studies have been done. Until then, Phen-Fen will remain off the market.

The Puzzle Within the Puzzle

With Phen-Fen gone, millions of overweight people across the country and in Europe felt unhappy and betrayed. The Holy Grail of weight loss—the key to the fat-storing switch—had been handed to them, then snatched away. The search was on to find a replacement. Phen-Fen showed us that throwing the switch was possible, but we had to find another way to do it.

Phen-Fen seemed to work for nearly everyone, so it was only natural to go looking for another drug, or combination of drugs, that we could give to every patient who walked in the door. We tried Meridia and Orlistat, but neither showed the spectacular results we obtained with Phen-Fen.

Slowly, however, I began to notice something about my patients that started me thinking in a new direction. Although they all shared a similar problem, being overweight, their eating habits and the way they experienced hunger fell into four very distinct categories.

What was going on?

Here are profiles of four typical but very different patients. See if you recognize yourself among them.

ANNE MARIE

Ann Marie is thirty-eight years old, 5'5" tall, and weighs 180 pounds. She came to my office, quite distraught, telling me, "Dr. Rivas, I've tried everything to lose weight and just can't do it. I've read every diet book and tried every program. I'm always hungry and dieting. Also, when I eat I either don't get full or it takes a couple of hours for the fullness feeling to come. By then I'm absolutely stuffed and feel sick. Sometimes I don't get full at all, and an hour or two after a meal, I start eating all over again. In fact, I have to practically starve myself to lose anything at all. I even tried to exercise four times a week for the past month, but haven't lost one single pound. My family doctor told me that I am eating more than I admit and I just need to pull myself away from the table and exercise more, but I swear, I'm *always* dieting! My metabolism must be dead. I have no energy so exercising is very hard, and sometimes I even feel slow mentally."

MARY ANN

Mary Ann presents a very different picture. She's a forty-two-year-old woman who has tried "absolutely everything but just can't lose weight." She has actually been exercising an hour a day and has been very careful about her fat consumption. Unfortunately, all her efforts have met with no success at all. She states quite emphatically that her appetite is normal and that she doesn't think she feels unusually hungry most of the time. She does have very significant cravings for candy, cake, pies, and chocolates, however. "I know, even at the time, that I shouldn't eat them but I do anyway." She also admits to compulsive eating. This means that she eats even when she's not hungry, usually in response to stress, depression, loneliness, or boredom. On occasion, she may binge eat, or eat to great excess. She can be moody, often showing symptoms of PMS, and sometimes, especially during the winter, she becomes severely depressed.

CARLA

Carla presents yet another picture. She's a fifty-year-old who's tried not only diets and exercise but also prescription medications such as phentermine and various natural weight-loss products as well. "I've lost about ten pounds and that's it," she says. She also feels listless and has no particular interest in doing anything. "I'm not sure if I'm depressed or just not enthused about anything. Nothing seems to excite me." She complains of craving fatty food and chips, but sweets aren't really a problem.

Susan

Susan was 5'6" tall and weighed about 220 pounds. Her appetite was extremely well controlled and she wasn't overeating, but her weight remained high. "This is so frustrating," she would tell me. "For breakfast I'm eating a bagel with nothing on it; for lunch, a half sandwich of fat-free turkey; and at dinner, I'm having fat-free pasta with a salad. For an evening snack I'll have a few pretzels. That's it for the entire day. It's impossible that I'm not losing any weight!"

Here's what fascinated me: The symptoms of each of the first three women were typical of someone who was lacking in a particular neurotransmitter. Anne Marie's constant hunger was a classic symptom of norepinephrine depletion. Mary Ann's bingeing indicated that her serotonin levels were obviously out of whack. And Carla's listlessness and lack of interest in anything was a textbook picture of someone suffering from a dopamine deficiency.

Susan was another story. She was obviously *not* a case of neurotransmitter imbalance. What struck me about her daily fare was that it was comprised mostly of carbohydrates. I had

News from the Brain Chemistry Front

Although we're very familiar with the effect serotonin, nor-epinephrine, and dopamine have on appetite, scientists are learning more about the brain chemistry of obesity every day. Within the past couple of years, researchers have discovered even more neurotransmitters (substances in the brain that cause cells to send an electrical message) that may affect the way you eat and gain weight.

Two of them, called *hypocretin 1* and *hypocretin 2,* are located in the hypothalamus, a tiny part of the brain that controls food intake. They're similar in makeup to a hormone called *secretin,* which controls acid production in the stomach.

Although we're not sure yet exactly how these two substances control weight gain, their location in the brain tells us that they almost certainly have a profound effect.

run into this kind of patient before, even during the Phen/Fen days. Susan is a classic example of what I call the *carbohydrate-sensitive* individual. These people will not lose weight until their diets are very starch and carbohydrate free. I find this condition in about 5 percent of my patients. One man who came to me gained 55 pounds just by adding pretzels to his diet after having lost 70 pounds. Another lost 65 pounds over three months by greatly limiting carbohydrate intake. (He had lost only 5 pounds during the previous three months, despite eating very, very little.)

Back on Track

If weight loss was a matter of targeting neurotransmitter imbalances, then throwing the switch would be easy. We already had safe and effective tools for doing that: Some were prescription medications, but others, which were just as effective, could be purchased without a prescription at any vitamin or health food store! And the best news of all was that people would be able to lose weight with no effort whatsoever. Just throw the right switch, and the pounds would disappear on their own. It was all simply a matter of figuring out which type of weight gainer you were.

I found that I could figure out each patient's type with about three minutes of conversation. And once I knew that, I could give them tools more powerful than Phen-Fen for getting down to a healthy, normal weight.

Identifying Your Type

Here are the questions I ask each of my patients on her or his first visit. Answer them as accurately as you can, and you'll know your own type when you're finished.

PART 1

1. Do you have a large appetite? Do you almost always feel hungry? Can you eat almost anything in sight?

2. Do you have a hard time getting full? Does it feel like you can just keep eating and eating? Is the feeling of fullness delayed, so that you've already eaten too much by the time the feeling of fullness occurs? Do you ever feel full at all? Do you even know what it means to be full?

3. How is your energy level? Do you feel tired frequently and blame your exhaustion on your weight?

4. Do you suspect that you have a slow metabolism?

5. Do you have trouble with motivation?

6. Do you have problems focusing on any one task? Are you scattered? Do you have symptoms of attention deficit disorder (ADD)?

7. Does your weight just seem to climb for no apparent reason or change of lifestyle? Are you out of control? Are both diet and exercise programs ineffective?

If you answered "yes" to most of these questions, then you are a norepinephrine-deficient brain chemistry type. Call yourself an N-Profile.

Part 2

1. Are sweet cravings more of a problem than hunger? Is chocolate your weakness? Are cravings a significant problem at ovulation or menses?

2. Are you a compulsive eater? Do you eat in response to various stresses, i.e. loneliness, boredom, anger, happiness, etc.? After you eat, do you ask yourself why you just ate?

3. Do you binge eat? Do you find yourself eating very large quantities of food at one sitting? Do you eat so much at one time that you get nauseated?
4. Are you obsessed by food? Is food on your mind through most of the day and does it sometimes even awaken you at night? Are you up in the middle of the night eating? Are food thoughts driving you nuts? Is food too great a priority in your life?
5. Do you get depressed, moody, and irritable? Do you suffer with PMS? Do you have seasonal affective disorder or fibromyalgia? Do you suffer with migraines?
6. Do you have a family history of alcoholism, depression, or PMS symptoms?

If you answered "yes" to these questions, then you are a serotonin-deficient brain chemistry type. Call yourself an S-Profile.

Part 3

1. Do you continue to have cravings for salty or sweet foods even after various medications have been tried?
2. Do you not enjoy life? Are you generally a "down" person?
3. Do you have an addictive personality? Do you need drugs to get high and forget your problems?
4. Are you easily distracted?
5. Do you experience sexual dysfunction?

If you answer "yes" to these questions, then you are a dopamine-deficient brain chemistry type. Call yourself a D-Profile.

PART 4

1. Are you unable to lose weight despite excellent appetite and craving control?
2. Are low-calorie diets ineffective?
3. Does exercise cause no weight loss at all?
4. Do medications fail to help you?
5. Do you tend to eat mainly carbohydrates such as breads, pasta, fruits, etc.?

If you answer "yes" to these questions then you're carbohydrate sensitive. Call yourself a C-Profile.

That's all there is to it! Now you have all the basic understanding you'll need to throw the switch and start losing weight.

4

N-Profile: The Universal Type

f you have an N-Profile, you're in good company. Epinephrine deficiency is by far the most common weight-loss challenge I see in my practice. But N-Profiles aren't the only people who suffer with the problem. *Everyone* who is overweight, to some extent, needs to raise his or her norepinephrine level. That's why *it's important that you read this chapter no matter what your profile*.

If you're lucky enough to be an N-Profile—the simplest and easiest of the disorders to treat—raising your norepinephrine level is the only step you'll need to take to lose weight. If you have a different profile, however, you should also read all chapters that specifically apply to you.

Joanne's Story

When Joanne first came to my office, she was twenty-seven years old, 5'4" tall, 190 pounds, and beginning to feel as if her difficulty in losing weight would drive her over the edge of sanity.

When she sat down across from me in my consultation room, she looked distraught and tired.

At one time or other, she told me, she had tried practically every fad diet program on the market, from those that offer weekly weigh-in meetings to those that restrict you to mail-order food—which they're happy to provide at a premium price. None of them worked. Her hunger was too strong.

"I can't stop eating," she said. "I'm always hungry and my appetite is unbelievable. I don't even know what being full feels like."

To make matters worse, she wasn't burning up many of those extra calories through physical activity. She felt too tired to exercise. Sometimes, in desperation, she forced herself to ignore her insatiable appetite and restrict her food intake to levels that would frighten a fasting monk. Unfortunately, that didn't work any better than the fad diets had.

She felt she had come to the end of the road where her weight was concerned, but, in fact, she hadn't. She had simply, finally, made the right turn.

The N-Profile's Profile

Literally thousands of people have come to my office reciting almost exactly the same tale of frustration and disappointment.

Often a patient will confide that she has other family members who suffer from similar weight problems or, just as telling, from attention disorders. She may have been quite thin for most of her life, then watched in horror as her dress size suddenly began to increase in an uncontrollable way. Her energy level slipped into the doldrums, a fact she attributes to her weight and poor metabolism. She is clearly depressed, and she even complains about having difficulty concentrating and focusing.

Below are the main symptoms to look for. If you have two or more of them, then the norepinephrine level in your brain is probably out of balance.

Hunger

As with Joanne, the most prominent symptom of the typical N-Profile person is increased appetite. Often she'll feel hungry through most of the day, but she'll feel absolutely famished in the late afternoons and evenings. Typical N-Profile hunger demands "real foods" rather than junk foods.

Insatiability

The N-Profile person does not always overeat but always wants to. She may complain that she "never feels full" during meals and doesn't know when to stop eating, so she'll just choose some arbitrary moment to quit the table. She may never feel full, or the feeling may hit her two to three hours later, when she'll find herself feeling absolutely stuffed. The feeling that you're full is called *satiety*. So if you can't achieve that feeling, you're literally insatiable.

Cravings

The N-Profile person may also have cravings but most often for starches, like breads and pastas, rather than sweets, and the feelings are occasional rather than constant. Some people mistake cravings for hunger, but there is a difference. A craving is a very strong desire for a particular food that cannot be satisfied by anything else. Hunger is more general and non-specific.

Exhaustion

N-Profiles may have low energy levels, but this has nothing to do with low metabolism. It's because their brain norepinephrine level is low. Norepinephrine is very similar to adrenaline, often called the "fight or flight" transmitter. Both substances are potent mental and physical energizers, so it's not at all surprising that a person with an N-Profile will often feel "blah."

Those Norepinephrine Blues

Many people complain that they wake up tired and can't get themselves moving all day. They often suspect, erroneously, that their thyroid is out of whack. Other people seem "okay" in the morning but generally burn out with fatigue as the day goes on. These are the folks you'll see taking afternoon naps.

All of this fatigue can come with some jitteriness and shakiness, which is often blamed—again erroneously—on a drop in their blood sugar or a hypoglycemic event.

Amazingly, these symptoms almost always completely resolve after raising the brain's norepinephrine levels. The person feels great throughout the whole day and evening. All of this suggests that their symptoms were actually from low norepinephrine levels and not from low sugar levels or hypothyroidism at all.

N-Profile

SYMPTOMS

- Hunger
- Insatiability
- Cravings for starchy foods
- Depression
- Exhaustion
- Attention deficit

Attention Difficulties

N-Profiles often, but not always, complain they have poor focus and concentration. One of my patients is a business executive and owner of a very large company. He told me how difficult it used to be for him to run his business effectively because his mind was always wandering. Because his ability to concentrate on a single issue was poor, at times so was his memory. After his norepinephrine levels were restored to balance, he was like a different person. Now, his business is booming, and, as an added bonus, his interaction with his family has improved. He is a much more patient listener and much more efficient at everything he does. If this sounds like ADD, that's because it is. What we commonly refer to as ADD is most certainly nothing more than a neurotransmitter deficiency, which can be easily corrected in most instances. When there is a coexisting weight problem, it is easy to correct both at once.

Depression

The N-Profile person may experience some depression—not usually profound but bad enough to interfere with daily life. Often she won't realize how "down" she really is until she's thrown her norepinephrine switch and notices at once how light her spirit has become.

Nature's Treatments

There are some natural supplements that can be extremely effective at turning off the hunger switch, as long as they're used properly, which means taking the proper dosage, at the right times of day, and in the most effective combinations.

A POWERFUL COMBINATION

The most effective—and most controversial—natural treatment for weight loss is the combination of ephedra with caffeine. Most often this appears on the label as ma huang with guarana.

Before you shake your head, wag your finger, and say, "But all the reporters on the six o'clock news are warning us NOT to use ephedra," consider this: Ma huang has been used safely by the Chinese for thousands of years as an energizer and weight-loss enhancer. People in many other parts of the world also have used it.

When large numbers of Americans began to discover the benefits of this ancient secret, however, the inevitable hap-

Why Do We Need Green Tea?

Ephedra, on its own, won't do much to help you lose weight. That's because the body produces enzymes that quickly break down norepinephrine in the system, so as soon as you produce a little more, it rapidly goes away. The catechins in green tea, however, stop those breakdown enzymes from being released. That leaves the norepinephrine to do its job of helping to control fat metabolism and increase calorie burning (*thermogenesis*). The caffeine in the tea has shown to be effective at increasing thermogenesis as well.

pened. Reports of problems began to surface, as they do whenever large numbers of unsupervised people start ingesting any substance that's stronger than a sugar pill. Even commonplace foods, such as shellfish, peanuts, and chocolate often cause allergic reactions that are sometimes so powerful they can become life threatening. So it would come as no surprise if ephedra turned out to be a danger to the public health. But is it?

For years now, the FDA has attempted to limit the use of ephedra products because of adverse event reports, but those attempts have never been successful. The reason: No one has been able to prove a causal relationship between the adverse effects and ephedra.

In fact, researchers from Harvard University and Columbia University have just finished a six-month-long trial on the safety and effectiveness of ephedra. What did they find? First, that it works. At the end of the trial, subjects who had been taking a combination of ephedra from ma huang and caffeine from kola nuts had lost a significant amount of weight, lowered body fat, and reduced hip measurements. They had also lowered their levels of dangerous LDL cholesterol, raised levels of beneficial HDL cholesterol, and reduced blood sugar levels. Of course, they also experienced side effects. Heart rate and blood pressure went up very slightly in some patients, although not enough to be dangerous. Some others complained about dry mouth, heartburn, and insomnia. All in all, however, the results showed herbal ephedra to be extremely safe and effective.

Then what about all those "adverse events" reported to FDA? Are people simply imagining things? Upon close inspection, it appears that most of the reported problems arose when consumers deliberately overdosed themselves, ignored warnings about drug interactions and preexisting medical conditions, or in some other way misused the substance. To complicate matters even further, the FDA employed very poor technique in gathering their data—which is why Congress has rejected the FDA's request to limit sale of the substance.

In one case, for example, the FDA reported that an eighteen-year-old male committed suicide while using ephedra. It would be easy to make the assumption that ephedra caused him to suffer a depression that lead to his death. However, an autopsy revealed that the young man had both ephedrine and *codeine,* a controlled narcotic, in his blood. And no data whatsoever were offered on the source, dose, or length and frequency of the man's use of the ephedra.

In another case, a thirty-year-old female died in the middle of the night in a car accident. She had been speeding at ninety miles per hour in the wrong direction up a one-way street. She ran a stop sign and hit a tree. An autopsy showed ephedrine and caffeine in her blood, so, of course, they had to be the culprits behind her risky behavior. Except that the same autopsy showed the presence of pseudoephedrine (an over-the-counter antihistamine) in her blood as well as an alcohol level of .212 percent!

In other cases, one woman claimed ephedra caused her Norplant contraceptive device to fail and was thus responsible for her pregnancy. Another blamed ephedra for excess nose and body hair.

The Final Word on Ephedra

For years, a nonprofit consumer group called Public Citizen has done its best to influence the U.S. government to take ephedra products off the store shelves. The results of the Harvard-Columbia study, however, have foiled their efforts, at least for the time being. Tommy G. Thompson, secretary of Health and Human Services, has declared that the government will not limit the sale of ephedra unless further studies show the need to do so.

Given what we now know, ephedra, when taken as directed, seems to be a safe and effective product. However, like many over-the-counter products, it's not for everyone. People with an overactive thyroid, heart disease, untreated high blood pressure, anxiety disorder, prostate enlargement, diabetes, or glaucoma shouldn't take it. Neither should anyone under the age of eighteen, pregnant women, or nursing mothers. And never take ephedra if you're already taking an MAO inhibitor or decongestants.

To put all this in better perspective, in 1999 there were 25 reported significant adverse reactions out of 3 billion servings of ephedra. This is an incredibly low incidence. By those statistics certainly almost any ingested substance—including peanut butter or oysters—is more dangerous. My patients have used ephedra/caffeine with great success and have had no serious problems.

As Effective as Prescription Medication

There is no question that ephedra/caffeine (EC) is effective at turning off the hunger switch. A very well designed, controlled study in Denmark of subjects using EC over a six-month period showed an average weight loss of 37.4 pounds. Another study concluded that EC is more effective than the old weight-control drug Redux™.

EC is also unique in that it encourages the body to burn fat rather than muscle, unlike most diets, which cause significant muscle wasting. Furthermore, EC seems to target belly fat, which is the most dangerous form. And unlike some medications, EC does not seem to lose its potency over time. It remains very effective after months of daily use.

EC has another significant advantage beside weight loss and its beneficial effects on serum cholesterol and blood sugar levels: It improves concentration and energy.

Its mechanism of action is rather clear. Ephedrine increases release of norepinephrine in the brain. Caffeine inhibits the breakdown of norepinephrine. So norepinephrine levels go up, the brain chemistry has a better balance, the thermostat goes down, the switch goes off, and weight loss ensues.

How to Use EC

Dosage is very important both for effectiveness and safety. The dose of ephedra should probably not exceed 48 milligrams per day, though there aren't many studies to support this statement. This is my experienced opinion. I also much prefer tablets, as they can be broken in half. Because the Columbia-Harvard study concluded that ephedra was safe to use for six months, I would suggest that after a similar time period you take a break from ephedra for a month or two, just to be on the safe side.

Ephedra usually comes in the form of the Chinese herb ma huang, but it may also simply be labeled as ephedra. I prefer my patients to use yet another form, called *country mallow,* although it's much harder to find. Country mallow contains very low doses of ephedrine alkaloids, substances similar to ma huang, which are also used in common, over-the-counter allergy medications.

Start with one-half of a 12-milligram tablet at 11 A.M. and 4 P.M. If you tolerate this dose well and you haven't noticed any change in your feelings of hunger, you can go up to one tab twice a day. If you need to, you can go higher, but max out at two tabs twice a day.

Side effects, which are similar to those of caffeine, often appear after the initial dose but diminish after continued use. They include mild nervousness, insomnia, agitation, and a slight rise in blood pressure. You're far less likely to experience these side effects if you use country mallow rather than ma huang. Men with enlargement of the prostate may notice a decrease in urine flow, so they may not want to use ephedra. People with heart disease, untreated hypertension, anxiety disorders, or prostate enlargement should avoid ephedra. If you find the speed at which your heart beats has increased, make sure your family doctor sees you on a regular basis to monitor you (losing weight under a doctor's care is a good idea in any case). Finally, if you have an overactive thyroid gland (hyperthyroidism), do not under any circumstances use ephedra or any product containing ephedra alkaloids. Always check with your doctor before taking any over-the-counter weight-loss product.

Medications that should not be taken with ephedra products include MAO inhibitors (i.e., Nardil™, Clonidine™, and Yohimbine™). If you're taking decongestants, stop using ephedra immediately if you notice any unusual side effects.

It's important to note that ephedra alone is not very effective in causing weight loss. You need to combine it with a caffeine product such as guarana or my current favorite, green tea extract.

Green tea contains two main active ingredients, catechins and caffeine, both of which lead to norepinephrine release. The catechins in green tea help to rein in an enzyme called *COMT,* which breaks down norepinephrine. The caffeine does the same thing to an enzyme called *phosphodiesterase,* which again leads to higher norepinephrine levels.

Recent studies set the effective dose at 50 milligrams of caffeine and 90 milligrams of catechin taken three times a day with meals. The catechins work best in the form of *epigallo catechin gallate,* but unfortunately, containers don't always carry this information. I recommend taking 200 milligrams of green tea extract twice a day.

Green tea has another benefit, by the way: It may reduce the risk of heart attack by 45 percent.

TYROSINE CAN HELP

A much lesser known but very effective natural product is the amino acid L-tyrosine. Combining it with ephedra can

Where to Find L-tyrosine

L-tyrosine is a naturally occurring food component that balances brain chemistry by raising norepinephrine and dopamine levels. It seems beneficial for improving mental performance, reducing stress, overcoming addictions, elevating mood, and increasing sex drive. In conjunction with other agents, it can also turn back the thermostat in the brain, flip the hunger switch, and reduce weight.

One way to help increase the L-tyrosine levels in your brain is by getting more from the foods you eat. Here are the top picks for tyrosine-rich foods:

✓ Wheat germ
✓ Ricotta
✓ Cottage cheese
✓ Pork
✓ Chicken
✓ Turkey
✓ Duck
✓ Wild game

reduce appetite by 50 percent more than by using ephedra alone.

This intriguing amino acid raises both dopamine and norepinephrine levels. It has been found useful in treating attention deficit problems, addictions, fatigue, narcolepsy, depression, and sexual dysfunction.

Its effects on reducing stress are rather striking. Studies done by the U.S. military show a significant reduction in combat fatigue and battle stress among those taking L-tyrosine supplements. In yet another study tyrosine increased cognitive performance, improved mood, and sped up the reaction time of subjects.

Its effect on appetite and brain chemistry regulation is maximized when it's combined with other weight-loss substances. I have combined country mallow with green tea extract and tyrosine with very good results. Doses of 500 milligrams to 2,000 milligrams per day are quite safe and effective. As with almost everything else, it shouldn't be given with MAO inhibitors.

5

S-Profile:
The Depression Connection

Serotonin is another, very powerful neurotransmitter that your brain uses to control mood, emotions, aggressiveness, sleep, and appetite. A low level can do more than cause you to gain weight; it can also plunge you into the deepest, blackest depression.

We've known about the connection between being overweight and depression for a long time. In fact, the first side effect researchers noticed when they began studying fluoxin (Prozac) was that it sometimes caused weight loss. This drug, of course, is aimed directly at raising serotonin levels in the brain.

The S-Profile's Profile

S-Profiles, people who are serotonin deficient, are the second most common type of weight gainer. Very often they share some characteristics with N-Profiles, but their serotonin symptoms are far more powerful. Here's what to look for:

Cravings

If you have an S-Profile, then you know the meaning of the word craving, especially where sweets are concerned. Pastries, cookies, candy seem to reach out and touch you. Chocolate—oh, that wonderful chocolate—holds more allure than gold. Otherwise, you may have a perfectly normal appetite. You don't feel hunger is your constant companion, and meals make you feel full, as they should. And you probably have no problem with any food type other than sweets.

Cravings are not a minor problem. In fact, they can be completely overwhelming. One of my patients described how she used to awaken in the mornings surrounded by empty candy bar wrappers. She had no idea she had even eaten them during the night.

Compulsive Eating

Another common symptom of the S-Profile patient is eating without hunger, most often in response to stress or uncomfortable emotions. You may find yourself eating when you're depressed, bored, anxious, or lonely. You may not even realize that you're eating. S-Profile people often munch unconsciously. Then after they've finished, suddenly become aware that they've consumed the equivalent of an entire meal—a meal they really didn't want.

Food Obsession

Sometimes an S-Profile person just can't get food off her mind. In fact, food is all she thinks about. This then leads to irrational, ritualistic eating behaviors, over which she seems to have little or no control. This is similar to an obsession with cleanliness that leads to compulsive hand washing. People will wash their hands to the point of scrubbing off layers of skin, even though they know that what they are doing makes no sense and that it is hurting them. They just cannot help themselves.

Binge Eating

This is an extremely exaggerated form of compulsive eating and/or craving. You may eat an enormous quantity at one sit-

Just What Is Serotonin?

Like other neurotransmitters, serotonin is a substance that passes messages from one brain cell (neuron) to another. The brain needs these transmitters because its cells don't actually touch one another. Serotonin levels seem to have an effect on mood, anxiety, arousal, attention, aggression, and thought. As important as its function is to the brain, however, serotonin is present in other parts of the body as well. It's present in blood vessels, which it constricts, and in the walls of the large intestine, where it increases the motion that moves food through that part of your digestive system. In fact, only about 2 percent of the total serotonin in your body is in your brain.

ting and feel quite ill afterward. Episodes may be either common or rare, but they tend to come and go.

Depression

It's not unusual for an S-Profile person to have a history of depression or to have used antidepressant medication. Often, people will complain that their depression is linked to their weight, but actually it's a separate issue. The good news, however, is that you can clear up both problems at the same time.

Anxiety and Panic Attacks

Anxiety is a feeling of vague uneasiness or apprehension over nothing in particular. It can be mild and tolerable or quite severe. Sometimes it can generate panic attacks. Severe and often disabling, these attacks can overwhelm you with feelings of pain, shortness of breath, sweating, shakiness, and nervousness.

The S-Profile at a Glance

SYMPTOMS

- Cravings
- Compulsive eating
- Food obsession
- Binge eating
- Depression
- Anxiety and panic attacks
- Phobias

Phobias

If you've ever had an irrational fear of anything at all that stops you in your tracks and seems to completely immobilize you, then you know the meaning of the word *phobia*. Whether you're afraid of heights, crowds, small spaces, or spiders, the panic and paralysis are the same and are due largely to a deficiency of serotonin.

Nature's Treatments

Several natural products will elevate serotonin levels, but to maximize their effect, you'll need to use them with norepinephrine-raising supplements.

The best supplement for raising serotonin levels is tryptophan, an amino acid that consumers once used extensively as a sleep-inducing agent. Unfortunately, in 1989 a fatal outbreak of a rare autoimmune disease, called *eosinophilia-myalgia syndrome* (EMS), was associated with the use of tryptophan. All of the evidence clearly pointed to a contaminant in the processing plant of one Japanese manufacturer. However, in a perplexing decision, the FDA has banned its use as an over-the-counter supplement ever since.

Prior to this contamination, people all over the world used tryptophan for many years without incident. Since there doesn't seem to be a problem with tryptophan itself, it's unclear why it wasn't allowed back on store shelves once the contamination issue was resolved. As of 1996, you can once again buy tryptophan, but to do so you need to bring a prescription to a compounding pharmacist (one who mixes compounds).

Effective doses range from 500 milligrams to 2,000 mil-

Tasty Tryptophan

The FDA may have taken tryptophan off drugstore shelves, but you can still find it at your local supermarket. Plenty of delicious foods can add tryptophan to your diet. Generally turkey and milk are good sources. Here is a list of other foods that contain tryptophan:

- ✓ Wheat germ
- ✓ Cottage cheese
- ✓ Pork
- ✓ Luncheon meat
- ✓ Duck
- ✓ Avocado
- ✓ Ham
- ✓ Eggs
- ✓ Almonds

ligrams a day. For the best effect, you can take tryptophan at night and the amino acid L-tyrosine in the morning.

If you don't want to go to the trouble of getting a prescription filled, however, you can purchase a product called 5-HTP (5-hydroxytryptophan) over the counter. 5-HTP comes from the seeds of a plant, the griffonia tree, which is native to Africa. People in Ghana and the Ivory Coast use the seeds to calm their children. Many Western doctors have also used it successfully, and some studies have proven its effectiveness in treating depression as well as obesity. I know of physicians who also use it for fibromyalgia and allergies. It's even used to help control anger, irritability, and anxiety.

One study looked at weight loss among overweight diabetics who took 5-HTP in very large doses (250 milligrams three times a day). The subjects who used the supplement lost an average of 4.6 pounds more than did the subjects who were given sugar pills. Another study showed a 5 percent weight loss over twelve weeks among subjects who took a dose of 200 to 300 milligrams before meals.

The results of both studies were affected by a common side effect of the supplement if taken in high doses: nausea. I have also seen a fair amount of nausea associated with this supplement, especially among patients who are taking the antidepressant drug Effexor, so I would avoid that particular combination. Nausea tends to go away by the second week of using 5-HTP.

I prefer a sublingual (under the tongue) spray of 10 milligrams per spray, which bypasses the GI tract and thereby avoids any nausea. The spray works in about two minutes, as compared to fifteen minutes for a capsule. The spray can be used on an as-needed basis and is especially effective in curbing sweet cravings.

As with any substance that raises serotonin, to make a significant impact on weight loss, you should use 5-HTP in combination with N-Profile agents, such as ephedra-caffeine products. Take them as you normally would, and use the 5-HTP spray as needed throughout the day. If you can't find the spray, try using the supplements. Dr. Michael Murray, the author of a book on 5-HTP, gets an average weight loss of a pound a week using 50 to 100 milligrams in supplement form three times a day, twenty minutes before meals. He also finds it useful for depression and fibromyalgia. If nausea becomes a problem, ginger tea may help.

Yerba Maté

Lately, I've come across a tea called yerba maté that could be a very real breakthrough for both weight loss and weight-loss maintenance. Yerba maté comes from South America and traditionally has been used as an overall stimulant and tonic, but it has multiple other health benefits as well.

A recent study out of Denmark initially brought yerba maté to my attention. In it, some forty volunteers were asked to take capsules containing the tea for forty-five days, other study participants were given a placebo. Those taking yerba maté lost an average of almost 2 pounds per week—with no adverse reactions! Of equal interest, they were able to maintain their weight loss for twelve months, at which time the study concluded.

Yerba maté seems to possess several mechanisms that account for its remarkable success, possibly the most prominent being what we refer to as *delayed gastric emptying*. This condition means that after taking in food the stomach remains full for a longer period of time and sends a message to that effect to the brain, which results in less food intake later. The phenomenon was actually confirmed by sound-wave, or ultrasonic, testing of patients.

Yerba maté also contains other interesting, effective components, such as xanthines, saponins, triterpines, and theophyllines, which probably have a direct effect on the brain. Xanthines and theophyllines both increase levels of norepinepherine, but through a different mechanism than that used by ephedra. Yerba maté also has a less stimulating effect than ephedra, with most people experiencing no jitteriness. And there's some evidence suggesting that the methylxanthine component directly stimulates the burning of fat.

As a side benefit, yerba maté is rich in several minerals, including calcium, magnesium, potassium, and copper. In addition, it has even been reported to lower LDL, or "bad," cholesterol, and seems to have a positive influence on cardiovascular health overall.

6

D-Profile: The Root of All Pleasure

Researchers have a theory. They believe—at least many of them do—that every pleasurable feeling we have, from the excitement of sex to the ecstasy of listening to a symphonic masterpiece, funnels through the dopamine system in the brain. Dopamine, like norepinephrine and serotonin, is a potent neurotransmitter, and the message it transmits from cell to cell is pleasure. One of its other jobs is closely related: It not only allows you to feel pleasure, but it drives you to seek it out.

The more dopamine you make, the better you feel. Of course, the opposite is also true. The less you make, the more blah your day is likely to be. If you're too low on the stuff, that last symphony or romantic encounter felt . . . well . . . okay, but not really wonderful. In fact, if you're low on dopamine, everything feels sort of okay but never any better than that.

If that sounds like a description of your own experience, then you may have a D-Profile.

Portrait of a D-Profile

Sometimes the easiest way to identify a person with a D-Profile is by her responsiveness to treatments for norepinephrine and serotonin depletion. In other words, it's a process of elimination. Or perhaps she started to lose weight on those other treatments but then suddenly stopped until a treatment that raised her level of dopamine kick-started her fat-burning engine into overdrive.

If you take a close look at yourself, however, you should be able to recognize your own D-Profile by the common characteristics listed below.

Depression

The neurotransmitter dopamine is responsible for the "natural highs" that people experience. The high of winning a sports

D-Profile at a Glance

SYMPTOMS
- Depression
- Addictive personality
- Sexual dysfunction
- Specialized cravings

competition or getting a good grade in school or a promotion at work all originate with dopamine.

Therefore, those who have a depleted supply of this transmitter may feel generally down or depressed or just blah. They have a hard time getting motivated or enjoying the pleasures of everyday life. This could lead to the extreme of a rather severe depression.

Addictive Personality

Alcohol, tobacco, and many dangerous "street drugs" can stimulate dopamine release, which is what makes them so addictive. People who are especially sensitive to these substances probably have an unusually strong "dopaminergic" response because their basic levels are low. This is most likely the foundation in the brain for the so-called addictive personality, often the hallmark of a person with a D-Profile. If you find that you can easily make a habit of taking substances that give you pleasure, or if you have a strong family history of addictions, then you may find that raising your dopamine levels will help you lose weight.

Sexual Dysfunction

Since dopamine is what allows you to experience the pleasure of orgasm, a low level may lead to sexual problems. You might experience delayed orgasm or even the inability to have an orgasm at all. Or you may simply find that your sexual desire has dwindled like a candle flame running out of wick.

Unfortunately, people often live with this kind of problem for years without recognizing its cause. They may blame themselves or their partners. Or sometimes their partners may be very angry with them for their lack of sexual interest or response.

Specialized Cravings

Strong desire for either fatty or salty foods is another D-Profile signpost. They tend to love bacon, sausage, steak, and other high-fat treats. A craving for starches is also common. So these people may show a strong desire for potato chips, corn chips, or salted, buttered popcorn.

Nature's Treatments

If you've kept up at all with the news in the world of natural medicine, you've heard about a particular amino acid called

The Obesity / Cocaine Connection

Cocaine, carbohydrates, and fatty foods may all have something in common: They may all increase the level of dopamine in the brain, thereby leading to addiction in the case of the drug, or obesity in the case of the foods.

Cocaine is the most powerful dopamine-raising agent we know of. By dramatically increasing the level of dopamine available to synapses in the pleasure center of the brain, the *nucleus accumbens,* it rewards the user with tremendous rushes of pleasure that "teach" the cells to hunger after more cocaine. Carbohydrates, while not nearly so powerful, can have a similar effect. When we consume lots of rice or pasta in response to a craving, we may simply be reacting to signals sent by brain cells, requesting higher levels of dopamine. Wellbutrin™, SAM-e, phenylalanine, and L-tyrosine all give higher levels but keep them within a safety zone—and they don't bring a lot of fat or calories with them.

The Satiety Substance

In 1998, researchers at the Yerkes Primate Research Center of Emory University published the results of a study that revealed yet another connection between cocaine and appetite. While looking at the effects of cocaine on the brain, scientists discovered a new neurotransmitter that seemed to regulate the feeling of fullness you get when you've eaten enough. They called the substance Cocaine and Amphetamine Transcript (CART) because it seemed to increase in the brain of rodents who had been given cocaine. The researchers discovered that when the substance was present in high levels, the rodents lost their appetite. When amounts were low, their appetite increased. These results helped explain why cocaine and amphetamines had such a dramatic weight-loss effect on users. In the future, these studies may help scientists to develop safer and more effective drugs in the treatment of obesity.

SAM-e (S-adenosyl L-methionine). It's become a popular remedy for arthritis and depression. If you're a D-Profile, it can also be very effective in helping you lose weight, if you use it in combination with N-Profile and S-Profile supplements.

Researchers have found that L-methionine raises dopamine, norepinephrine, and serotonin. It comes as a supplement and is also found in certain foods such as sunflower seeds.

If you take SAM-e, it's important to use B_6 along with it to prevent the SAM-e from converting into homocysteine, a substance that can increase your risk of heart disease. As an antidepressant, methionine has proven as effective as many prescription medications in clinical trials. It appears to be very safe, even at large doses, especially when taken with vitamin B_6. You can take 1 to 3 grams of methionine per day.

SAM-e can be expensive. Another amino acid, phenylalanine, is a more economical alternative. Phenylalanine, a "precursor" of tyrosine in the body, elevates both dopamine and norepinephrine and helps to keep them in balance.

In addition to weight loss, phenylalanine has been used effectively for depression at 200 milligrams a day and is better absorbed than tyrosine. It can be a rather effective pain reliever and can be used for PMS symptoms. It's highly concentrated in meats and cottage cheese. You can take up 8 grams per day in supplement form.

People can't take phenylalanine if they have PKU, phenylketonuria, which is a rare illness affecting 1 in 40,000 people.

7

C-Profile: When Pasta Is the Problem

Medical science is full of mysteries. We don't really understand how some people spontaneously recover from incurable diseases, why some people become mentally ill, or what triggers a person to start putting on weight by so much as tasting a slice of white bread. Yet these things happen.

Yes. There are people whose brain chemistry is so sensitive to the effects of carbohydrates that they absolutely will not lose any significant amount of weight unless they severely reduce their carbohydrate intake. This is the essence of the C-Profile.

What are carbohydrates? To put it simply, starches and

sugars. Rice, beans, bread, pretzels, corn, potatoes, white sugar, brown sugar, honey, pasta—some of our very favorite foods—all fall into the category.

The C-Profile's Profile

The C-Profile weight gainer is typically the most difficult to diagnose. About one in five of my patients shows an hypersensitivity to carbohydrates, so it's not a terribly unusual condition. What makes it so difficult to diagnose is that it displays no easy-to-spot symptoms. Generally, I'll make the diagnosis simply by excluding all other possibilities.

Here's what generally happens. On her initial visit, a patient—we'll call her Julie—will seem to present the symptoms of a mixed type. Maybe she has a strong appetite, some cravings for carbohydrates, and her mood seems generally blah. I'll first give her a combination of weight/appetite-reducing agents such as the supplements in this book (or if she prefers, safe and effective medications) to turn off cravings, decrease appetite, and increase fullness.

At this point, the typical person would easily lose weight because her brain chemistry is in balance and her thermostat is pushed back. But in Julie's case, the weight seems to cling to her stubbornly, despite an absence of cravings, compulsive eating, or ravenous appetite. No combination of medications or supplements leads to weight loss. There is only one conclusion left: She has a type of extreme carbohydrate sensitivity that makes it extremely easy for her to gain weight and difficult for her to lose it.

Carb Addiction?

You don't have to be a "carbohydrate addict" to have a C-Profile. Maybe you swoon over sweets and pasta, or maybe you don't. The point is not how much you crave these particular foods, but rather how your body reacts to them. What seems to happen is that carbohydrates, even in small amounts, keep C-Profile people from burning their body fat as fuel.

Jean-Pierre Flatt, Ph.D., a leading researcher in energy metabolism and body weight reduction at the Department of Biochemistry at the University of Massachusetts Medical School, has shown how this occurs. It has been a long-held belief among scientists that the body readily transforms carbohydrates into fat, which it then stores to use as fuel. Flatt has demonstrated that, to the contrary, excess carbohydrates are not easily converted to fat but instead are stored as glycogen, a substance the body burns in preference to fat. In an interview for the newsletter "Obesity Research Update," Dr. Flatt was asked, "Are carbohydrates important to weight control?" He responded, "Yes. Carbohydrates determine the amount of fat that is burned. The more carbohydrates you eat, [the] less fat you burn. The less carbohydrates you eat, the more fat you burn. A person can burn 150 to 250 grams of fat per day if carbohydrate intake is restricted to 50 grams or less. This is roughly one-third to one-half a pound of fat per day."

So we know that the presence of glycogen in the body will turn down the controller in your brain that tells you to burn fat as if it were a dimmer switch. What we don't know is why, in some people, a small amount of glycogen suddenly signals the switch to turn off altogether.

Treatment

I start my patients for the first two weeks on a very restricted carbohydrate intake, just to see what kind of response I get. If a patient loses 5 to 10 pounds over this period, I have my confirmation that carbohydrate sensitivity is the problem.

Essentially, meals during this time consist of nothing but eggs, bacon, meats, poultry, seafood, diet drinks, cheese, cream, nuts, broccoli, cauliflower, and salads. If the approach proves successful, the person can slowly increase her carbohydrate intake until she's consuming 30 to 50 grams per day.

Assuming she continues to do well, I'll keep her at this level and offer her a low-carbohydrate menu and recipe book as well as various tasty food and shake supplements. The rest is up to her.

If she wants to remain thin, she'll have to follow this regimen religiously for the rest of her life. Of course, anyone who has ever tried sticking with a high-protein and very-low-carbohydrate diet knows how difficult a challenge it can be. This kind of diet is especially tough on women, who generally tend to like carbohydrate foods more than men do. In fact, Julie might very well find the task impossible. That's why, to quiet her cravings and appetite, it is absolutely necessary for Julie to continue taking her natural supplements. It will also help if she allows herself plenty of variety in the foods she eats and rewards herself with an occasional "vacation" from the diet.

Unfortunately, it's not clear what the long-term ramifications

The Body Resists

Even if you love steak, fish, and chicken, giving up or lowering your daily carbohydrate consumption isn't easy to do. In fact, your body may naturally resist all of your very best efforts. In May 1998, researchers at Ohio State University's Department of Food Science and Technology presented findings at a meeting of the American Society of Nutritional Scientists that suggested that's exactly what your body *will* do.

In an ingenious experiment, scientists gave twenty-five male college students a Carnation Instant Breakfast™ every day for three weeks. Here's the catch: Three different types of shakes were given. Some of the men got whole-milk shakes, some got skim, and others got skim with sugar added. Each week, the type of shake each man got was changed. Neither the researchers nor the subjects knew who had which kind of shake at any time.

The results showed that over the long term, no matter how much fat or carbohydrate was added to or subtracted from his breakfast shake, each man would unconsciously compensate at other meals the rest of each day, so that by evening, his totals would always be the same.

The results suggest that, just as there's a set point in the brain that determines body weight, there's also a set point for the amount of carbs and fats each person consumes in his or her daily diet.

of this type of high-protein diet are. There is concern that too much protein may be dangerous to the kidneys, but that concern is based on theory, not research. Some studies do suggest that, since early man was primarily a hunter and meat eater, he should be able to adapt himself healthfully and naturally to this way of nourishing himself, but they're far from conclusive.

To Shake or Not to Shake

In general, I don't see the point in replacing regular meals with special, designer diet foods such as protein shakes because they quickly become monotonous and people stop using them. In the case of C-Profile people, however, protein drinks can have their place.

Some people get bored with eggs, sausage, and cheese after a while, so drinking a shake now and then actually adds some variety to their meals, which is very appealing. In fact, I've treated a few brave souls who jump-started their new low-carb eating plan by consuming five protein shakes a day for the first two weeks and after that, one shake before each meal to further curb their appetite.

Shakes can also be useful in getting those last 5 to 10 pounds off—the ones that always seem so difficult to lose.

C-Profile at a Glance

SYMPTOMS
- Mixed symptoms from the other profiles
- Failure to respond to drugs or natural supplements
- Quick weight response to lowering or raising of dietary carbohydrates

Obviously, shakes shouldn't be the centerpiece of your diet over the long term. They simply don't offer the nutrition that the human body needs. I would also recommend that anyone temporarily using shakes as a primary food and calorie source take a multivitamin every day.

8

Guess What Doesn't Work!

Check out any pharmacy, supermarket, or health food store, and you'll find enough weight-loss products, both prescription and over the counter, to make you dizzy. And, of course, don't forget the various programs, approaches, and devices offered through infomercials, magazines, and alternative practitioners.

So what works and what doesn't? We've already talked about the most effective tools you can use to turn off your hunger switch. Is there any value at all to any of the other "pounds-off" promises the marketplace offers you every day?

Here's what we know about some of them.

Acupuncture

Most people these days have some passing familiarity with this ancient form of healing from China—or, at least, have heard of it—but few are aware that it may actually be an effective weight-reducing technique.

Acupuncture represents a holistic approach to health, a balancing of all the opposing forces within you. Hair-thin needles are inserted along "meridian points" on the body. Meridians might best be described as places where energy can be stopped, diverted, or increased.

To some Western doctors, all this sounds more like poetry than medicine, but there is no doubt that acupuncture has proven effective in the control of both acute and chronic pain. In China it is even used in place of anesthesia during surgery!

There was some initial promise when a study in Taiwan followed forty-five subjects with diet, exercise, and acupuncture. They lost an average of 9.7 pounds after two months. But obviously, the diet and exercise could have given that modest degree of weight loss over such a short period.

I have had patients tell me that ear acupuncture makes mildly spicy foods tastier. But I have never seen acupuncture cause weight loss, and some controlled clinical trials have all proved negative.

In all fairness, I have seen remarkable improvements in pain relief and control of anxiety. It is therefore conceivable that combined with medications, acupuncture could control stress eating in conjunction with the drugs. This study has not been done and maybe should be. Multiapproach therapy is almost always preferable to the single approach. So acupuncture could still be useful as part of a multimodality treatment for obesity. Forget it as the sole regimen.

Amphetamines

Forty years ago, these drugs represented the gold standard for weight-loss medications. They are powerful appetite inhibitors, but they are also dangerous and addicting. People who use them over an extended period of time often become restless and nervous. Many develop the "shakes," a chronic and noticeable trembling of the hands. Insomnia is common. Overdoses can cause depression, psychosis, and death. Enough said?

Aromatherapy

This treatment is based on using the essential oils of certain plants, which are inhaled, diluted, or added to a bath. The inhaler is the most convenient form and is prepared by mixing 15 drops of bergamot oil and 10 drops of fennel oil in a small airtight container. The oils are mixed very gently and then used as an inhalant for hunger control.

Dr. Alan Hirsch has done most of the research on this therapy. He studied 3,000 subjects who inhaled green apple, peppermint, and banana odors whenever they experienced hunger or cravings. Those who responded best were medium- to large-frame people and were chocolate cravers. The subjects lost an average of 1 pound per week over six months. It is theorized that the odors work directly on the appetite center of the brain. People who suffer from asthma or migraine headaches shouldn't use these inhalers.

I've never tried this form of treatment, so I can't comment on it fairly. There seems to be some promise here for certain individuals. The weight loss is slow but reasonable. It doesn't work for everyone, and it's likely that a tolerance would develop over time. Again, I wouldn't suggest using it by itself, but rather alongside other approaches.

Chromium

You've seen the ads; you've heard the claims:

"Lose the fat, keep the muscle."

"Lose unwanted fat while reshaping your body to a leaner, trimmer, firmer physique."

"Improves your metabolism so your body relies more on using stored fat and less on proteins . . . resulting in more muscle and less fat."

"No dieting, no exercise required."

"Melts the fat away."

"Plays a key role in reducing fat through better appetite control and increased metabolic rate."

"Dramatically reduces body fat, lowers cholesterol, builds leaner muscle mass."

"Works by making your body more sensitive to the hormone insulin."

If all or even some of these claims are true, then chromium must be a candidate for the weight-loss miracle of the century. Chemically, chromium is a trace mineral, a substance that exists naturally in the human body in minute amounts. It's certainly necessary for good health, but should we encourage people to use large doses in supplement form? Is it safe and effective?

I first became interested in chromium when another physician called to confer with me about one of his patients who had come to me for help with weight control. The physician said he was impressed with the results his patient had achieved on our program, and wondered if we had ever used chromium as a natural appetite suppressant. He had used it for years to better control blood sugar levels in diabetic patients, and he claimed it also helped them with losing weight.

I try to be open minded to new approaches to weight control, and I am normally very receptive to the idea that vitamin and mineral supplements can have great benefits for the human body. I take daily megadoses of antioxidant vitamins every morning to help prevent cancer and heart disease. I even believe that alternative therapies make sense in the management of some patients.

When I heard that chromium might help some of my patients, I immediately began collecting all of the literature on chromium that I could find.

The theory went like this: Chromium transports sugars and amino acids, which are the building blocks of proteins and muscle, into the cells of the body. Therefore, if you take lots of chromium, you will build lots of muscle, which will then burn lots of fat for fuel. I immediately became suspicious. The "more is better" theory hardly ever proves true where the human body is concerned. It's like saying that if a little fat in your diet is necessary and good for you, then lots and lots of fat must be even better.

Most of the early work on chromium was done by Gary

Evans, a chemist who works in the nutrition field. He developed a process to synthetically manufacture chromium picolinate and did two field studies on weight training. In the first, he gave 200 micrograms per day of chromium picolinate to a group of college students who were training with weights. He reported that after six weeks, the students showed an average 3.5-pound increase in muscle mass, while a control group taking a placebo showed slightly less than a pound of increase per subject. The second study, carried out on college football players, used the same method and, according to Evans, yielded similar results.

Criticism of the studies has been vehement. Hank Lukaski, research leader at the U.S. Department of Agriculture Human Nutrition Research Center, stated in April 1994 at the North Dakota Academy of Science, "For young men trying to maximize their strength—or anyone else—chromium picolinate has no effect on building muscle, reducing body fat, changing body composition, decreasing weight or increasing strength."

Robert Lefavi and colleagues, in the *International Journal of Sport Nutrition,* have criticized Evans's scientific method and questioned both the effectiveness and safety of chromium supplements. Unfortunately, only a few studies other than Evans's have been done. In one, football players from the University of Massachusetts team showed no change in body composition after nine weeks of taking chromium supplements and doing intense conditioning exercises every day. In another study, thirty-five healthy men reported the same results after eight weeks of chromium use, although researchers did note that the subjects were excreting five times the normal amount of chromium in their urine.

A study in 1996 showed slightly more positive results. People taking 200 to 400 micrograms of chromium per day

Let the Buyer Beware

Here are some of the weight-loss scams and frauds that the Federal Trade Commission is warning consumers against:

- ✓ Any program that promises you'll lose 30 pounds in thirty days
- ✓ Skin patches
- ✓ Shoe insoles
- ✓ Fat blockers that purport to prevent fat absorption (with the exception of Orlistat)
- ✓ Fat "magnets" that purport to flush fat out of the body before absorption
- ✓ Diet teas
- ✓ Products containing glucomannan, chromium picolinate, hydroxycitrate, guar gum, fat emulsifiers, cellulose/fiber, and ox bile extracts
- ✓ Fiber tablets
- ✓ Bee pollen
- ✓ Laxatives
- ✓ Electrical muscle stimulators
- ✓ Passive-motion exercise devices
- ✓ Hunger-suppressing ear cuffs
- ✓ Acupuncture devices
- ✓ Body wrappings, belts, or girdles
- ✓ Any of the 111 over-the-counter substances the FDA has declared not safe or effective for weight loss

showed an average loss of 4.2 pounds of fat over two and a half months. If these results actually show what chromium can do, there doesn't seem to be much cause for celebration.

Fiber

Chromium isn't the only over-the-counter substance currently marketed as a miracle cure for obesity. Products containing high amounts of bulk fiber have also enjoyed a lot of fanfare. They're supposed to fill you up, and because fiber isn't stored or metabolized by the body, you won't gain any weight. Cellulose and other food fibers actually make you feel more full, but the effect is only temporary. Soon you'll find yourself facing the old cravings again. By the way, there is no evidence to support the claim that fiber stops the body from absorbing fat or that it speeds up metabolism. It's all hype that exploits the desperation of people who are in genuine need.

Although neither chromium nor fiber seems to be of much help in losing weight, other "natural" substances and approaches have shown promising results.

Chitosan

Chitin is the fiber found in the outer shells of soft-shelled fish, such as shrimp and lobster, and insects. Recently, it has been used in the manufacture of a fiber supplement, Chitosan, and touted as a weight-loss product.

The manufacturer's claim is that Chitosan will absorb twelve times its own weight in fat from the food you eat and pass through the body undigested, taking the unwanted fat with it.

I've seen no substantial evidence to support the claim. Animal studies show minor positive effects from the product. It does seem to lower fat absorption slightly, by about 8 percent, and works better when supplemented with vitamin C, but it also lowers protein and calcium absorption. If you take this product, be prepared to boost the calcium and protein in your diet or with supplements.

No study has shown this product to have any effect on weight loss, and the cost may be prohibitive.

Citrimax

For centuries in Asia, people have used an extract from an evergreen plant, called the *Malabar tamarind,* to season their food. The extract has a sweet, acidic taste and seems to make people who use it feel more full and satisfied after a meal. The scientific name for the extract is *hydroxy citric acid,* or HCA. It is marketed in this country under the name Citrimax™.

Theoretically, HCA works by diverting carbohydrates and fats into the liver for storage as a substance called glycogen rather than into cells for fat storage. It was promoted as an appetite suppressant and cholesterol reducer. There was some initial enthusiasm and hope for this product, but it has been a dismal failure when put to the test in clinical trials.

A study in 1998 at St. Luke's/Roosevelt Hospital in New York City showed HCA to be ineffective at causing weight loss in humans at the standard dose of 1,500 milligrams per day. The group taking the placebo actually lost more weight than those on the HCA did! In August 1999, results of a very well-designed study from the University of Colorado showed that HCA does not cause fat or calorie burning. Another study, reported in June 1997, of fifty overweight women who took HCA as well as caffeine showed no significant weight loss after six weeks.

More significantly, studies done on animals by the drug manufacturer Hoffman-La Roche showed that HCA caused testicular atrophy. They didn't dare to proceed to human studies.

In summary, the product is ineffective, and if you're a male, possibly even hazardous to your health. I'd avoid it!

Essential Fatty Acids

While it's true that too much dietary fat can be dangerous, it's also true that you need to eat some fat to be healthy.

Essential fatty acids are fats that come from plants and fish. They come in two varieties: omega-6 (linolenic acid) and omega-3 (linoleic acid). You get plenty of omega-6 in the vegetable oils you use when you cook, make salads, and bake. Omega-3 isn't as plentiful. You find it only in fish oil and oils made from canola, soy, and flax.

For good health, you need to consume about three times as much omega-6 as you do omega-3. If you go on a very-low-fat diet and don't get enough of these nutrients, your skin will eventually become very dry, and your hair will start to fall out. It takes a while, sometimes two to three months, for these effects to appear, as your body stores EFAs in plentiful amounts and it takes you some time to use them up.

In extreme cases, a patient deficient in EFAs will form gallstones, a very serious condition. If there is no fat whatsoever in the diet, a person will die within two weeks. So whenever you're on a diet, it's a good idea to supplement with EFAs.

On the plus side, some recent evidence shows that EFAs can enhance fat burning and increase metabolism. They can also lower cholesterol levels and raise calcium levels in the body.

I supplement my patients' diets with oil of evening primrose (1,300 mg) twice per day. I also suggest they take one capsule of flax oil (1,000 mg) every day. This combination gives them plenty of omega-6 and omega-3 oils in the proper ratio, and prevents any of the harmful side effects associated with low-fat diets.

Hypnosis

Hypnosis is another popular alternative for weight control. I've had a few patients swear by it. Unfortunately, even when it works, the results are temporary at best.

The general idea of hypnosis is to induce a mental and physical state of relaxation through suggestion, which will then allow you to gain better control of your eating behavior.

I believe that in those for whom it's successful, the relaxation phase is the result of a rise in brain serotonin levels. It's very much like taking a low dose of a serotonin-raising drug. Both approaches can lead to less compulsive eating, but in both cases, the results are only temporary unless combined with a norepinephrine agent, like phentermine or ephedra/caffeine. Remember, if only your serotonin level increases, you'll eventually *gain* weight.

Hypnosis may be valuable when combined with either natural or pharmacological agents to establish an even greater serotonin balance, which would, in theory, lead to better control of cravings, compulsive eating, and binges. However, I don't believe that this combination effect has ever been studied.

Herbs

Herbalists have recommended all kinds of plant therapies to help people lose weight. Unfortunately, most don't work. The following popular herbs seem to have little or no positive weight-loss effects, either among my own patients or among those involved in any of the clinical trials I've examined: St.-John's Wort, kelp, gotu kola, ginkgo, garcinia, parsley, dandelion, corn silk, juniper berries, seaweed, chickweed, fennel, and ginseng.

Orlistat

This drug, sold commercially as Xenical™ keeps you from absorbing much of the fat from the food you eat. Clinical trials show that people have lost 10 percent of their body weight with regular use. Among my patients, however, the side effects of the drug—which include fatty diarrhea, cramping, fecal incontinence, and oily discharge—were so severe that I stopped recommending its use. Whatever happened in the clinical trials, I've never known anyone who tolerated using the stuff long enough for it to be effective.

Slim•Fast ™

This is a low-calorie meal-replacement milk shake that actually seems to work for some people. However, it has two drawbacks: First, it contains 40 grams of carbohydrates and 35 grams of sugar, making it a disaster for people with a C-Profile. Second, while many people find the taste pleasant, drinking it every day can become extremely monotonous, and the overall low-calorie diet of which it is a part is very hard to comply with for longer than a few weeks.

9

Keeping the Switch
in the Off Position

Many, if not most, people who take the supplements outlined in this book immediately begin looking forward to the day they can stop taking them. As soon as they get their weight down to a normal level, they think that they will be "cured" and they can stop taking pills.

I wish it were so, but for most patients, unfortunately, it is not. True, a few lucky individuals will find they can maintain healthy eating habits even after they've gone off their medications, but most will require very low maintenance doses for the rest of their lives.

Don't Take It Personally

Once again, it is important to remember that being overweight is a chronic, medical condition, not a character flaw. I would not expect a patient with elevated cholesterol to show normal lipid levels in her blood if she stopped her medications; neither would I expect healthy blood sugar levels in a severely diabetic person who suddenly discontinued his insulin shots. In the same way, I don't expect most obese patients who go off their Hunger Switch program to continue enjoying freedom from food obsessions.

It is the word *freedom* that confuses most people. How can you be free if you're dependent upon supplements?

Where your weight is concerned, the answer is simple: You can use weight-control agents to help free you from overeating, or you can continue to overeat and be free from the use of weight-control agents. It's sort of like saying you can work to free yourself from poverty, or you can remain poor to free yourself from the need to work. The choice is yours.

A Horse of a Different Color

Most people don't realize that losing weight and maintaining the lost weight are two very different animals. Losing weight requires an adjustment of brain chemistry, which leads to an adjustment of the brain thermostat controlling your weight. Once the body reaches its new setting, your weight will level off and won't go any lower.

Why? The brain is always in full control of where it wants

your weight to be. The final number has nothing to do with ideal body weights, insurance company charts, or BMI indices. Your brain doesn't care about charts. It only cares about balancing its own chemistry.

This Is How We Do It

Compared to losing weight, maintenance is somewhat easier, but it requires a serious, long-term commitment. Your job now is simple: Keep your brain chemistry in proper balance forever.

You may find that you can stop supplements and maintain your weight for six months up to even two years. In fact, giv-

Nature's Fat Fighter

Two recent studies, one published in the December 2000 issue of *The Journal of Nutrition,* and the other presented at a meeting of The American Chemical Society in Washington, D.C., in August 2000, both confirm the fat-fighting effects of a substance that occurs naturally in meat, poultry, and dairy products called CLA (conjugated linoleic acid). About 3 grams of the stuff daily (1 gram before each meal), along with very light exercise, safely and effectively reduced the amount of fat people carried in their bodies while increasing the amount of muscle. When people were maintaining their weight, CLA helped to make sure that any pounds they gained back came in the form of muscle. So if you're determined to go off your medications or supplements, you might consider taking 1 gram of CLA with each meal, every day.

ing your body a vacation from these substances is probably not a bad idea. But at some point, your brain's chemistry will start to go out of balance again, and your weight will begin to make its way upward.

It's a frustrating situation, because it will happen without your changing your eating habits. You can even try to eat less, but your weight will continue to climb. In the end, it may exceed your initial weight. The reason for this is clear: Your brain chemistry is in full control, and it's telling you to store energy in the form of fat rather than burn it as fuel. Diet and exercise can't keep up with the new situation and inevitably fail.

So you have to keep taking the pills, just as if you were treating any other chronic medical condition such as hypertension, elevated cholesterol, diabetes, or depression. There is no cure, only control. The supplements will control your brain chemistry, which will in turn control your weight. Only genetic engineering or manipulation will actually cure weight problems.

Fortunately, the average person can maintain her new weight by taking her medications or supplements on Monday, Wednesday, and Friday only. If that doesn't work, try taking them every day, but cut the dose in half. It's that simple.

Exercise Can Play a Role

Although exercising doesn't do much to help you lose weight, it can have some value in maintenance. It will help to raise your metabolism and burn off any extra calories you may consume. However, exercise alone won't keep you at your ideal weight.

The problem is that the exercise has to be very strenuous, regular, and long term if it's to carry the burden of your entire weight maintenance. In the absence of medications, you would have to work out one to two hours every single day for life. Most people can't commit themselves to a lifetime of exercising on those terms. Sooner or later, circumstances interfere with almost any exercise program. It's a fact of life, and there is no point in preaching otherwise.

What About Vitamins?

Many people ask me about supplemental vitamins and/or minerals as part of an overall healthy eating pattern for life. Multivitamins are not very useful in my opinion. They give too little of each nutrient to be beneficial.

I prefer my patients to take significant amounts of individual nutrients. For prevention of heart disease, I recommend 400 to 800 micrograms of folic acid per day and 400 to 800 IUs of a mixed tocopherol vitamin E per day. For cancer prevention, 200 micrograms of selenium is an excellent choice. Several studies have shown a decrease in cancer risk by about 60 percent when selenium is taken. If you want B vitamins, then get a high-potency B complex with at least 100 milligrams of each B vitamin.

Some patients have told me that horse chestnut is excellent for fluid retention and edema. Black cohosh and soy isoflavones are both very good for hot flashes, which occur during perimenopause.

10

Choosing a Healthful Diet

You need to go on a diet. Now before you start groaning, let me explain. I do *not* mean an extreme weight-loss diet. Many of my patients have told me that on low-calorie diets they practically starved themselves to achieve weight loss, sometimes consuming as few as 500 calories a day. Not only is this kind of diet impossible to maintain, it's also unhealthy. Malnutrition becomes a real possibility, as does dangerously compromised immunity.

Fad diets are just as bad. Some of these can throw your nutritional intake badly out of balance, creating an entirely different set of problems. Most of the popular low-carbohydrate diets, for example, are loaded with red meat, which leads to a high intake of saturated fat, a known risk for heart disease, stroke, and vascular disease. A diet full of red meat also poses a very high risk of colon cancer. Furthermore, many meats are processed with sodium nitrites, which can increase the risk for several malignancies, including brain tumors. Diets extremely high in proteins may also lead to kidney failure.

To make matters worse, weight-loss diets work only in the short term. Over long periods of time, you'll probably

Why Calorie-Restricting Diets Don't Work

Research clearly shows that the number of calories you eat every day doesn't have very much to do with your weight. The HANES I Survey of 1971–75, for example, looked at the calorie intake and energy expenditure of over 20,000 Americans and discovered that thin people, on average, actually eat more calories than obese people. Other studies have reached similar conclusions.

Martha, one of my patients, is a typical case. She had been on one diet or another ever since she had been a teenager. All of them forced her to keep her calorie intake within the 500- to 1,000-calorie-per-day range. Not a nice way to live, but it did cause her to lose weight, on average about 40 pounds over three months. The problem was that after six months, she would gain 45 to 50 pounds back. After the cycle had repeated itself again and again, it became clear that not only had dieting failed to make Martha lose weight, it had actually caused her to gain some. Martha's story is a common one, and it's an object lesson for all of us: Losing weight is not about having the willpower to restrict calories.

Milk, the Weight-Loss Power Food

You've always thought of dairy foods as good for your teeth and bones, but did you know they can also help you control your weight? In April 2000, *Science News* magazine reported on research that describes how calcium influences the *agouti* gene, which determines whether you'll store the food you eat as fat or burn it as fuel. The study suggests that the average American woman doesn't consume enough calcium to make much of a difference, but if she actually consumed the recommended daily allowance every day—especially in the form of food rather than supplements—she could experience dramatic weight loss.

gain your weight back—and then some—even if you manage to maintain a low-calorie intake. There are sound reasons for this.

First, the body has an amazing capacity to adapt to and compensate for any dietary restrictions you subject it to. When you start to cut back on calories, you release certain hormones, such as the newly discovered peptide ghrelin, which then make you ravenously hungry. In other words, the hunger switch flips to the "on" position. That's why no one can stay on extreme diets for any length of time. It's just too hard. The hunger and cravings become overwhelming. Remember, food is necessary for life, so you can't just go cold turkey and eventually get over your desire to eat. You must constantly indulge to some extent, and with junk foods available on almost every street corner, you'll eventually give in to temptation and indulge in the unhealthiest, fattiest foods around.

Dieting also lowers metabolism, which means you burn less of the food you eat for fuel and store it as fat instead. All of this is the result of signals from your brain, which is genetically programmed to protect you from starvation. Remember, in the long history of the human race, we have had to adapt to some extremely harsh conditions, including famine. Fat storage is just the brain's way of getting us through tough times.

As you can see, dieting can't solve the basic problem. It can't change your genes or brain chemistry. It never addresses the root cause of weight gain. It treats the symptoms, but not the disease.

Here's to Your Health

Weight-loss diets don't make you lose weight but healthful diets do help you to stay healthy. The idea is not to cut calories back but rather to eat foods that will keep you well and avoid ones that can do you harm.

There are several key points in creating a healthful diet:

- It should be loaded with tasty food so that people can comfortably stay on it for life without significant modifications.
- It must be loaded with nutrients but low in fat and sugars, which are known to create health risks. According to the *Journal of the American Medical Association,* 300,000 people a year die from diseases associated with a high-fat diet, including heart disease, high blood pressure, stroke, cancer, arthritis, and multiple sclerosis.

- It can and should promote both weight loss and health at the same time.

The diet that seems to fulfill all of these criteria is the Mediterranean diet, so named because it represents the way southern Europeans living in the Mediterranean region normally eat. The foundation of this diet comprises seafood, olive oil, colored fruits and vegetables, and red wine. Each of these elements can make its own unique, healthful contribution to your daily fare.

Seafood

Recent evidence suggests that consuming cold-water fish, such as tuna or salmon, is very good for you. These fish—especially salmon—contain large amounts of omega-3 fatty acids, which are essential to our development and health and can only be obtained in the foods we eat. Omega-3s have been linked to lower levels of cancer and heart disease as well as improved immune function and healthier skin. Other sources of omega-3s are walnuts and wheat germ and, my favorite, flaxseed oil, which can be taken in 1 teaspoon of liquid a day or 4 capsules divided throughout the day.

Oils

Olive and peanut oils are monosaturated fats, a type of fat associated with low levels of heart disease and stroke.

Vegetables

Vegetables are not all created equal. Always look for the brightest and richest colors, which signify high levels of antioxidant phytochemicals, substances that eliminate dangerous "free-

Olive Oil: Miracle in a Bottle

Not only will olive oil help keep your cholesterol lower, but, according to some researchers, it will also give a boost to the supplements you're taking by actually helping you to burn off more calories! When you eat, the body either burns the calories you consume as fuel or stores them as fat. What decides which way the food will go? Chemicals called *coupling proteins* turn off the fat-storing switch and allow you to use up that energy in daily activities. In animal studies done in Spain, olive oil caused an increase in uncoupling protein production, which in turn caused a decrease in fat! This is great news for those of us who couldn't live without our bottle of extra-virgin.

radical" molecules that roam your body, causing damage to tissue. The best of these veggies are broccoli, kale, spinach, turnip greens, and peppers. Tomatoes are excellent sources of the cancer-preventing substance lycopene, as are ketchup and tomato sauces. One must be somewhat careful with fruits, as they can be very high in sugar. Again, the brightest, such as strawberries, blueberries, and raspberries, are best. In fact, blueberries are one of the richest sources of antioxidants known.

Wine

One or two glasses of red wine per day can be a healthful choice. A phenolic substance in red wine, called resveratrol, seems to lower LDL cholesterol levels in the blood. This may partially explain the so-called French paradox, which refers to the fact that people in France, who eat a lot of fat but drink wine regularly, tend to have low cholesterol levels. Remember, however, that wine may be somewhat weight inducing. You need to check this out for yourself and stop if it causes you to gain weight. Also, if you feel a strong urge to exceed one or two glasses a day, you may have a predisposition to alcohol addiction, so obviously you should cut the wine from your diet.

More Healthful, Delicious Foods

The foods above constitute the foundation of the Mediterranean diet, but you can certainly add others to make eating more interesting. Here are some great ones:

Nuts

Nuts are an excellent source of protein and are high in healthy monosaturated heart disease/stroke–preventing fats. One major study showed that women who ate nuts regularly for ten years were a third less likely than other women to suffer a heart attack. Particularly good are Brazil nuts (high in selenium), almonds, walnuts, and peanuts. Don't go overboard. It's easy to get too much of a good thing where nuts are concerned. Three or four nuts a day is plenty.

Breads

I'd limit breads to one serving per day and make sure that whole wheat is the first ingredient. Read the label and skip any bread that has sugar or dye added to it.

Dairy

Yogurt and cottage cheese have some health benefits but seem to behave like starches, so be careful. Milk is also a healthy choice, although you may want to purchase a low-fat variety. Eggs are extremely healthy and don't raise cholesterol levels! Foods high in saturated and trans-fatty acid raise cholesterol. You can eat eggs daily, and it's a great way to the begin the day.

Poultry

Chicken breast is an excellent, low-fat protein source. Obviously, avoid deep frying in lard and other saturated fats. Turkey is also a great choice and contains tryptophan, which will help turn off the hunger switch for S-Profiles. Don't eat the skin of any of these birds, as it's extremely high in fat. Also, watch your portions. Try to keep the portion of any fleshy, protein food (fish, poultry, beef) down to the size of a deck of cards or, at most, of your clenched fist.

Meat

Lean sirloin and other lean cuts of meat confer many health benefits and add to a well-rounded diet. Some research seems to suggest that grass-fed cattle produce meat that's as lean and healthful as game meat, which is very healthy indeed. If you live near an all-natural grocery store, you may be able to find these lean cuts.

The great thing about this diet is that it tastes good, offers a wide variety of choices, and is very health promoting. It's something you can live with while losing and maintaining weight loss. But, remember, the diet does not cause you to lose weight. It simply keeps you healthy while the supplements you're taking do their work.

When You Can't Go
Mediterranean

For heaven's sake, don't worry if you occasionally dine out at a restaurant or grab a meal at a fast-food place where you don't always know what's in the food. If you set a bunch of rules for yourself that make you feel miserable and deprived, you won't follow them for long. Remember, you're creating a new, healthy lifestyle, not a program that will last for only a few weeks or months. Make rules you can follow, and don't beat yourself over the head if you break them once in a while.

For example, if you find yourself eating at restaurants on a regular basis, just be reasonable with your choices. Use common sense. Check the menu or ask the waitress for low-fat selections. Grilled, skinless chicken breast, baked or broiled fish, pork loin, and even shrimp, lobster, and crab are delicious and healthy.

I remember the look of shock on the face of one of my patients, a young woman named Judy, when she told me that she still found herself wishing for chocolate cake on certain days. My advice to her? Eat chocolate cake. She immediately protested that she had always been warned to avoid this particular pleasure at all cost. If she had "always been warned," then chocolate cake must have always presented her with an unusually strong temptation. I asked her if she thought she could live the rest of her life without it. She sheepishly admitted that she couldn't imagine such a life. "Then why set yourself up to fail?" I asked her. "Eat the cake."

She still looked unsure. She wasn't so much concerned about her health as she was concerned about her weight. She was afraid that one taste of her favorite food would lead to a binge. I reminded her that as long as she was following the program for her profile and her hunger switch was in the "off" position, bingeing wouldn't become a problem.

It is precisely in this kind of situation—an uncontrollable craving for carbohydrate—that brain chemistry balancing agents do their best work. I knew that after eating a small slice of cake, she would feel satisfied and lose her craving, and I told her so. Neither would she be bothered by obsessive thoughts about food—any food!

I now have a patient who loves to go around telling people that she "has her cake and eats it too." Ah, well. I suppose eating less corn doesn't necessarily make you less corny.

Common Sense in Other Common Situations

What about eating out at the homes of friends or at those dinner parties your boss gives to show her employees what a great person she is or, worst of all, at wedding receptions, birthday parties, and anniversary celebrations? If the healthy choices available are limited, or if you find yourself facing a huge pile of food doled out by an overly generous caterer in the serving line, eat only a portion of it.

When you were a child, your parents may have ordered you to "clean your plate, down to the very last crumb" in a misguided effort to look out for your nutrition. Some teacher may have advised you to remember the poor, starving children in some third world country whenever you were tempted to "waste" good food. Well, you're no longer a child, and you need not follow bad advice from people with good intentions.

Some of you may have tried most of these dietary recommendations in the past but failed to follow them for any length of time. If you're on track with your profile plan, you won't fail this time. Why? Because your medications or supplements have rid you of your food obsessions and cravings. At last, you're free to take real control over your life and make choices that are about your health, not your weight.

11

Exercise to Feel Great

xercise won't make you thin. It simply takes too much physical movement to burn off more excess calories than you consume. In fact, it actually makes some people *gain* weight. If they exercise to the point of feeling hunger, it causes them to eat even more than usual.

"No problem," you say. "Exercise will speed up my metabolism, so I'll burn off any extra calories I take in." Don't count on it. While it's true that your metabolic rate will increase while you're exercising, and may even remain at that rate for several hours afterward, your body will then compensate by increasing its rate of food storage. This mechanism has developed over millennia of evolution to keep us from accidentally starving ourselves.

So why bother exercising at all?

While exercising may have nothing to do with weight loss, it has lots to do with health. The human body is built to move. It needs to work and play. It has muscles that push, muscles that pull, and a wonderful system for storing fuel for them to burn. When muscles are stressed by your pushing or pulling them harder or for a longer time than they're used to, they begin to break down. In response, your body builds even denser muscle so that next time you work out, you'll be better able to handle the workload. If you continue to stress your muscles by working them harder each time you exercise, the breakdown/rebuilding process will eventually leave you with a lean, muscular, athletic physique—something that losing weight by dieting alone can't give you.

Exercise has other great benefits, such as improving your self-image, self-confidence, and general sense of well-being. Strenuous activity can make you feel relaxed and good about yourself; it can give you a feeling of accomplishment, of having done a difficult task well. This effect is so strong that in study after study it has actually relieved symptoms of depression in people who are overweight.

Where your general health is concerned, exercise is the closest thing we know to a magic elixir. Statistics show significant increases in longevity among people who are even moderately fit. One Swedish study, for example, showed that female subjects who were most active between the ages of fifty and seventy-four were 33 percent less likely to die from heart disease. Other studies have shown that exercise also reduces the incidence of premature death from other causes—

colon cancer and breast cancer, for example. And research has also demonstrated that the obese and the elderly benefit greatly from exercise.

A Question of Motivation

An obvious question arises: If exercise is so wonderful, why don't we love to do it? Why don't we wake up in the morning eager to leap onto the stationary bike or to grab hold of a mean-looking set of dumbbells? Three words come to mind: *sweaty, painful, boring.*

Not everyone feels this way. Many athletes actually do look forward to exercise. So do ordinary folks who have made it part of their daily routine. Their muscles long to stretch and contract the way colts long to romp on the open range. But people who are out of shape, especially if they are also overweight, become disproportionately overstressed with even a small amount of movement. Their muscles are more like old nags than young colts, and chronic dieting has exhausted their systems. To make matters worse, they feel self-conscious and humiliated wearing workout clothes, such as shorts or tights, most of which are clearly designed to compliment lean bodies. All in all, the pain seems much greater than the gain.

Okay, then, you know it's good for you, but in your heart of hearts, you really, really, really don't want to exercise. You know that if you start a program today, in three months you'll get up one morning and say to yourself "I just can't do it this morning. I'm too tired. I'm too busy. I'm too whatever." You skip that day, and it feels good, so you skip another. And another. And pretty soon you're off your program. You were doing it because everyone told you how good it was for you and how it would keep you younger and stronger.

You had been telling yourself how wonderful it felt to be in better shape. And you were telling the truth—to a point. It did feel wonderful, but only after you had gotten the daily routine over with. Before and during, it felt lousy.

Okay. You really don't want to exercise. So don't. At least for now.

No, I'm not kidding. But I'm not letting you off the hook either.

Take Small Steps

As of today, let daily exercise become one of your long-term goals. See it as the finish line. For the moment, you are at the starting gate. Your first step will be to become less sedentary. There is only one unchangeable rule you must remember: For exercise to work, you must always push yourself to do just a little more physical activity than you're used to.

This doesn't mean giving up your desk job or forsaking your life as a homemaker for a career in day labor. It does mean looking for small ways in which you can expend a little more energy. They're easy to find.

Ask yourself some simple questions: Are there places I drive to that I could walk to? When I do drive, could I park a little farther from my destination to give myself the opportunity of walking? When I do walk, could I walk just a little faster? Are there times when I could climb steps rather than ride an escalator or elevator? Could I wash the dishes by hand sometimes rather than use the dishwasher? Can I use a push lawn mower rather than a self-propelled one? If I'm whipping eggs or mixing batter, could I do it by hand rather than use a blender or electric beaters?

There is only one caveat: Don't exercise so much that it makes you hungry. If you're taking supplements to reduce your hunger, then regularly participating in an activity that has the opposite effect is the last thing you want to do.

When Your Engine Starts to Hum

If you have been extremely sedentary, you'll find as you begin to move more that you'll want to move more, especially if you have lost 10 or 15 pounds through your *Hunger Switch* profile program. It feels good to use your muscles, and you'll find yourself growing impatient with sitting around and doing nothing. At this point, you may decide you want to begin a regular exercise program.

All kinds of questions will come up. What is the best program for me? Should I be jogging, lifting weights, doing aerobics, taking up tennis? How often do I need to exercise and for how long? Should I go out and buy expensive equipment? How about special clothing, like sweatpants and running shoes?

My best advice is to calm down. Take it slow. Low-intensity exercise is a perfectly good way to begin, and you're not ready for more yet. Begin with a fifteen-minute slow walk twice a week. As you feel more and more capable, you can gradually build up to longer treks.

If you're more comfortable indoors than out, or if the weather is a problem, try using a treadmill. Some studies have shown that it is the best indoor aerobic exercise you can do.

Take your walks just after a meal. If you exercise just before a meal, you'll dull your appetite a bit, but an hour later you'll rebound and become ravenous. It's not a good idea.

As you continue to become more fit, you may decide to go on to more strenuous exercising. If you do, bear a few facts in mind as you decide which type of program to undertake.

First, aerobic activities such as jogging or playing tennis will improve your endurance and the health of your heart,

Exercise for Seniors

Aging causes muscles to waste away. Elderly people can find themselves unable to do simple tasks, such as sitting up on their own or walking across a room. The only therapy that works for people in this condition is muscle building, so I took a group of ten people with an average age of eighty-five from a nursing home and conducted a weight-lifting class twice a week with them. We used dumbbells ranging from three to five pounds.

Within a few months, all ten people were all feeling an overall sense of greater strength and improved well-being. One woman gave up her cane as her upper-body strength increased. Another was able, for the first time in years, to make her way from her bed to a chair without the aid of a nurse.

but it won't change the way you look unless you're running marathons and burning up so many calories that the body can't compensate fast enough to put them back on. On the other hand, resistance exercise, such as weight lifting, will make you stronger and change your body's shape by building more muscle, but it may not do nearly as much for your cardiac health. Obviously, to get all the benefits possible from working out, you should do both forms of exercise as well as some stretching to keep you limber.

Reversing the Diet Effect

If you're like most overweight people, you've been on many diets, most of which severely restricted the amount of food you could eat. You lost weight, but what you may not have realized is that much of that weight loss was due to your body cannibalizing your own muscle tissue! The only way around this process is to build new muscle as the old muscle is used up.

A study from the University of Massachusetts demonstrates the point. The subjects were divided into four groups. Here are the results:

- The group that dieted alone lost an average of 9 pounds, but 11 percent of that weight was in the form of muscle.
- That group that dieted and did aerobic exercise lost an average of 10 pounds, but 99 percent of it was fat loss.
- The group that dieted and did strength training lost an average of 9 pounds, but all of the loss was from fat, and some muscle was gained in the process.

- That group that dieted and did both aerobic exercise and resistance training lost an average of 13 pounds, all of it in the form of fat, and gained 4 percent more muscle.

The result is clear: A combination of aerobic exercise and resistance training gives the best benefits. Walking and working out with very light weights is ideal.

Try to work up to two half-hour aerobic sessions and two half-hour resistance training sessions per week. If you're using weights, start with very light weights and exercise one muscle group per week (arms, chest, shoulders, back, etc.).

It's important to make frequent changes in your exercise program. For example, walk for a couple of weeks, then switch to a bike for a couple, then to a treadmill, then to a jump rope. This will keep your body from getting so used to any particular movement that it starts to get easy. You can also vary the intensity of your workout. Some days, walk a little longer or a little faster, or alternate from quick to slow pace as you go.

Watch What You Eat

Although you don't want to end up eating more due to exercising, neither should you cut your calories back in an effort to lose extra weight. Take your supplements and eat when you're hungry. When you exercise, you need fuel. If you don't have it, you'll quickly become fatigued and discouraged. Eat plenty of carbohydrates (vegetables, fruits, and grains) and protein, and keep your fat intake low.

The Big Picture

For convenience, here's a summary of the points you should remember about exercise:

- Exercise is better at helping you keep weight off than at making you lose it.
- A little activity is better than nothing. Start slowly; build up gradually.
- Overweight and fit is far better than overweight and out of shape.
- Resistance training with weights will build muscle and help you to keep a strong, fit body even while you're dieting.
- A combination of aerobics and weight training is ideal.
- A half-hour session, twice per week, of walking, biking, using a treadmill, or jumping rope is the goal you're shooting for.
- A half-hour session of weight training, twice per week, starting out with light weights and attacking only one muscle group at a time, is all you need of this type of exercise.
- Frequently vary the kinds of exercise you do.

Don't exercise until you're hungry, but don't cut back your calories either. Have faith in your natural supplement program to keep your food intake under control.

Don't be surprised if you find your weight going up a little. Muscle weighs more than fat, so trust your mirror more than your scale. If you really need numbers to make you feel good, ask your doctor to measure your fat-to-muscle ratio, or to recommend a place where you can have it done. This is sometimes done in a water tank, but usually it's just a matter of measuring your fat folds with a caliper.

12

Our Kids and Our Parents

Most of us would make any sacrifice to keep our children safe and healthy. We teach them not to talk to strangers, to look both ways before crossing the street, and to wash their hands before eating. We take them to the doctor for immunizations, earaches, and strep throat.

When they're a little older, we anguish over the dangers of drugs, sex, and violence. We're on constant lookout for anything that might threaten their young lives, and we would lay down our own to protect them.

Why then, do we ignore a serious and potentially catastrophic problem that affects the lives of a fourth of our kids?

What am I talking about? The fall edition of the *Archives of*

Pediatric and Adolescent Medicine reported that we now have twice as many obese children as we did ten years ago. One child out of every four is dangerously overweight. Many of these kids will go on to become obese adults. If a child is seriously overweight when he's ten to thirteen years old, he is six to seven times more likely than other children to have the same problem for the rest of his life. Even those who manage to lose their excess fat by the time they reach maturity aren't out of the woods. Obese children will suffer a greater risk of illness and premature death over the next fifty years of their lives, no matter how thin they become as adults.

No one is sure why obese children tend to become obese adults or, if they don't, why they suffer greater risks to their health. We have, however, identified some factors that increase their risk of obesity and some that do not.

Birth Weight

Many things affect how much a child will weigh at birth: Did the baby come before or after the due date? A child gains an ounce per day in the womb during the last month of pregnancy. How big was his mother? Genetics plays a significant role. Did the mother smoke during pregnancy? Smoking seems to cause lower birth weight.

One factor that has only a minor role to play is the amount of food a mother eats during pregnancy. Her body will keep the extra calories for itself rather than passing them on to her child.

As long as a baby falls within an average, healthy range, 5.5 to 9 pounds, birth weight is considered normal. Even at

Fat Television

Dr. William Dietz of the Harvard School of Public Health has discovered an interesting risk factor for children being overweight. There is a direct correlation between the number of hours a child sits and watches television and the degree to which he or she is obese.

Some of the reasons for this are obvious. Watching television is sedentary. People tend to consume more junk food as they watch. Advertisements for food may cause people to head for the refrigerator more often.

But Dr. Dietz has offered another, more subtle, reason: Watching television induces a trancelike state that may slow down the metabolism! The explanation that makes most sense to me is that this trance is like the hypnotic state, which raises serotonin levels without raising norepinephrine—a surefire way to gain weight.

higher weights, concern is more for complications during delivery than for any health problem the baby may be carrying. And there is no correlation whatsoever between what a person weighs on the first day of his life and what he will weigh on the twenty-first anniversary of that day.

In fact, that correlation doesn't occur until adolescence. It is the ten- to thirteen-year-old for whom we are most concerned.

Fat Cells

The total number of fat cells a person develops from age ten to thirteen may have something to do with the problem, but even this is controversial. Most people will end up with 120 to 160 billion fat cells in their bodies by the time they reach adulthood. Usually, that number is set during or just after adolescence. It would seem logical to conclude that the more fat cells you have, the fatter you will likely be.

Not the case. Fat cells are like deflated balloons. They take up very little space. Fill them with fat, however, and they'll blow up very big. So it's the size of the fat cells, not their number, that is significant. That means that you can have relatively few fat cells and still be obese. On the other hand, you can have many, many fat cells and never put on a pound of excess weight in your life.

What to Do

Modifying some of these risk factors may help children to maintain a healthy weight throughout their lives. Ignoring them, on the other hand, may lead to all sorts of health problems.

Seriously overweight children enter puberty sooner, have a shorter period of bone growth, and are at greater risk for high blood pressure, elevated cholesterol levels, orthopedic problems, and menstrual problems. Just as important, their self-image can become seriously distorted, leading to depression and worse. This is especially true among teenage girls. Eight out of ten, when polled, say they need to lose weight and would like to talk to a doctor about diet and exercise. Unfortunately, most are too intimidated to do so.

What Can We Do?

I have found over the past several years that weight loss in adolescents can be as difficult to achieve as it is in adults. Again, the problem is mostly due to genetic predispositions that lead to imbalances in brain chemistry. Diets and activity won't bring about permanent weight loss.

I must admit that this is a very tough problem. I don't yet have enough scientific data or experience to recommend the Hunger Switch approach for young children or for teenagers, but I believe it will eventually prove their most effective—and perhaps only—method of achieving long-term weight loss. Supplements and medications that are safe for adults are not necessarily safe for people who haven't finished growing and developing.

Until more studies have been done, your only option is to try traditional methods of weight control. If you can achieve any degree of success, you'll at least have done something to help your child. Here some approaches you can try.

- *Reduce fat.* Cut down on the fatty foods he eats, especially fast foods. This doesn't mean eliminating red meat and French fries from his diet altogether. Kids won't tolerate that. As in all things, moderation is the key.
- *Cut sweets.* You can reduce his snacking and desserts, but, again, don't be too rigid or strict. Try replacing

high-fat desserts with their low-fat counterparts, but remember that overindulging in anything that contains a lot of sugar, even low-fat foods, will put on weight.

- *Push protein.* Feed him more lean protein, fruit, whole grains, vegetables, and low-fat dairy products. It's not enough to get rid of the bad things in his diet. You have to replace them with good things.

- *Encourage exercise.* Get him to be more active on a day-to-day basis. Encourage him to climb stairs, do yard work, walk a little more, and anything else you can think of to keep him moving. Start him on an exercise program. Swimming, biking, running, and jumping rope are all good choices, but whatever the activity, it should be done four times a week in twenty-minute sessions. Kids find this kind of routine easier to follow when the entire family is involved, so parents and siblings should take the opportunity to get in shape as well!

Older Folks

Children, of course, are not the only people we love for whose care we are responsible. So, too, are our aging parents and grandparents.

For too long the attitude among physicians was that the health problems of the elderly didn't need aggressive treatment. They weren't going to live long anyway, so why risk making their lives miserable by changing their routines or making them swallow a bunch of pills that might have side effects?

To the credit of the medical profession, this attitude has changed, largely in response to research. Your family doctor now realizes that elderly patients benefit greatly from aggressive treatment of heart disease, diabetes, hypertension, and elevated cholesterol levels. Older patients also get great results from exercise programs, whether for improving aerobic capacity or for increasing muscle strength.

I'm convinced that elderly patients could enjoy healthier, longer lives if we also took an aggressive approach to helping them control their weight.

Of course, our concerns are the same as they would be in treating people in this age group for any other illness: drug/supplement interactions, coinciding illnesses, and dosage. Because older people are more sensitive in general to everything they ingest, elderly patients should start their regimen at the lowest possible doses and, if necessary, work gradually upward.

Consistent exercise will also help to vastly improve the quality of life for people in their later years. Building muscle will make them feel stronger, boost their sense of well-being, and make them more mobile. They'll also suffer from fewer falls and fractures. I wouldn't be surprised if their improved health allowed them to stop taking many of their other medications, which in turn would mean fewer side effects.

Overall, I look for a picture of much better health among our very young and very old as we bring their weight problems under control, but they are not the only population groups we need to single out for special attention.

13

Special Advice for Men

Men can use all of the information and advice in this book, but they're not likely to. In fact, it's hard to imagine a more uncooperative, unwilling patient than the average American male. Even if he's obviously ill, he'll resist doing anything about it until his symptoms get so bad they interfere with his work. Mention his weight to him, and you're lucky if he so much as loosens his belt a notch.

So if you're a woman, just how do you get your husband, father, uncle, or brother to pay attention to what's clearly a health risk as well as an appearance issue for him?

If a rash, fever, or elevated temperature won't drive a man to change his ways, how on earth do you get him to change just because his pants don't fit like they used to? This chapter is designed to help you do exactly that.

Moving the Mountain

If he's like most men, it is only when his weight begins to interfere with his day-to-day life by making him fatigued, sluggish, and short of breath after minimal exertion that he will actually consider seeing a professional. Even then, he may remain stubborn. It may take the onset of diabetes, arthritis, or some other weight-related illness to move him.

This, of course, is not an acceptable situation. Here's what to try.

Tell him what you see.
Make him aware that you notice he's overweight. He may not be paying attention to his shape, but he will if he knows you are. At the same time, let him know that you're not criticizing him but rather that you're concerned about his health. Point out that his apple-shaped physique (big belly, small hips), which is typical of the overweight male, has proven in study after study to pose far more of a health risk than does the pear-shaped physique (smaller belly, larger hips and buttocks) of the overweight female.

Share your successes.
If you've lost weight yourself recently or have done something else to significantly improve your appearance, let him know how good it makes you feel to look younger, healthier, and more attractive. Tell him you want the same things for him.

He'll want to look better for you at first, but as he begins to have some success with his weight-loss program, he'll also want to look better for himself.

List the professional advantages.

Gently point out that losing weight may help him in his job, especially if his work requires contact with clients or the general public. He may have already thought about this on his own. As a man grows older, he begins to realize that his younger counterparts have their eyes on his job or sometimes his clients. In a case such as this, a better appearance can mean the difference between success or failure in his career.

Tell him the benefits.

Point out that he'll feel better in general if he sheds his excess weight and gets into better shape. No one likes becoming short of breath and exhausted just from moving about the house or going up a flight of stairs. There's hardly a man alive who wouldn't prefer to have the energy, strength, and vigor to work all day, come home and play with his kids, go out for the evening to have a good time with the woman he loves, then come home with energy to spare for some bedroom romance.

The Upsides and Downsides of Being a Male

Men suffer a health disadvantage because of the way in which fat tends to collect around their abdomens rather than their hips and buttocks. On the other hand, their metabolism gives them a big advantage once they decide to get rid of that fat.

Because of his higher testosterone level, the average male will have significantly greater muscle mass than the average female. This greater muscle mass, in turn, allows him to lift heavier weights and work against greater resistance, which creates even more muscle mass. Since muscle cells are efficient fat burners twenty-four hours per day, all of this muscle helps him to lose weight more quickly than his female counterpart.

If men have all these advantages when it comes to losing weight, why should they be concerned about supplements?

There is one aspect of dieting at which men do not do well: portion control. What comes to mind when you think of a "man-size" meal? Enough food to feed a horse. The healthiest, leanest food in the world will put fat on you if you eat too much of it.

Thus, appetite control is a major issue for men. And the best way to control appetite, as we've seen, is to use the right tools to move the internal thermostat and turn off the hunger switch.

Body-Building Supplements

Men like to putter, fix, and improve. Very often, as soon a man begins to experience some success with a project, he immediately starts looking for ways to get even better results. This is usually the point at which he asks me about supplements that can help him boost his energy and muscle mass. These are the ones I'm usually asked about.

What's This I Hear About GHB?

Whatever you've heard, GHB is nasty stuff. In addition to its well-known use as a "date-rape" drug because it produces an alcohol-like inebriation, men have been using it as a body-building supplement. Bad move. It turns out that the stuff is highly addictive and leads to very serious withdrawal symptoms—serious enough to land many men in the hospital. And the symptoms, which include anxiety, insomnia, tremor, hallucinations, psychotic behavior requiring sedation and restraints, delirium, and loss of control of the autonomic nervous system, can last up to two weeks. In at least one case, withdrawal has lead to death. The same dangers hold true for GHB's chemical relatives, butyrolactone and butanediol.

DHEA

If he's done any research on his own, the first supplement he will ask about is DHEA (dehydroepiandrosterone), a steroid hormone that's supposed to do everything from curing cancer to reversing the aging process.

How many of these claims are true has yet to be seen. Not enough research has been done. We do know, however, that DHEA reduces body fat and raises metabolism, even when taken in doses as low as 10 to 25 micrograms per day. If supplements prove safe for human use, they could be a valuable addition to a weight-loss program . . . but that's a big "if."

DHEA occurs naturally in the body but in tiny amounts. No one knows what adding more of the chemical to the metabolic mix will do in the long term. My advice for now is to wait and see what the research eventually shows. If a man decides to use DHEA in spite of the risks, he should at least have his blood levels checked first, and talk over his decision with his doctor.

Testosterone

Supplementing with the male hormone testosterone also shows promise as an aid to men who are trying to lose weight and build healthier bodies. Testosterone will give more muscle and greater strength, increase your sex drive, and improve your memory. On the other hand, it can lead to aggressive behavior and prostate problems, so most doctors will insist on taking a blood level first, then supplement with doses based on the results.

We're still in the early stages of learning how to use testosterone effectively, but it shows real promise, especially for men over sixty years of age.

If a man has a well-rounded diet that includes plenty of different fruits and vegetables, it probably isn't necessary for him to take a daily multiple-vitamin supplement. However, I would suggest taking a good assortment of antioxidants. This is good advice for women, as well.

Antioxidants are substances that neutralize "free radicals," particles that roam around the body doing all sorts of damage at the molecular level and are responsible, at least in part, for aging and many diseases.

It's especially important to take antioxidants if you exercise vigorously. Tissue breakdown that occurs during exercise raises the level of free radicals in the body, so it's important to offset this effect with supplements.

Here's what I recommend:

- Vitamin E as alpha tocopherol: 400 International Units per day
- Selenium: 200 micrograms per day
- Pycnogenol: 30 milligrams per day
- Folic acid: 400 micrograms per day
- Zinc: 60 milligrams per day

It's better not to buy a general antioxidant that contains all of these ingredients, as it's nearly impossible to get the recommended doses of each substance into one or two pills. Buy them separately, but remember that more expensive doesn't necessarily mean higher quality. Shop for price. And don't forget to look over mail-order catalogues and sites on the World Wide Web. They are an excellent way to buy supplements at a reasonable cost.

14

Common Questions
with Uncommon Answers

A mong the many questions I've had from patients over the years are a few that come up over and over again. Some of them have undoubtedly occurred to you. I hope the discussions below will be helpful.

Q: Am I overweight because of poor eating behavior or heredity?

A: Both. Several studies have demonstrated conclusively that genetics exerts a strong influence over the tendency to gain weight. (See Chapters 1 and 2.) On the other hand, many other studies have shown that the amount of fat you eat also plays a role in determining how fat you become. This may seem contradictory, but it isn't. Heredity studies tell us that a person's genetic background will determine how likely it is that she will become obese, as compared to the rest of the population. Fat intake, however, helps to determine how fat any individual actually becomes. Heredity gives the odds; environment determines the real-life outcome. It's like a horse race: Theoretically the thoroughbred with the strongest lineage should win every race, but anything from track conditions to the temperament of the jockey can change the outcome.

Q: **If being overweight is a result of both heredity and environment, what does an imbalance in my brain chemistry have to do with it?**

A: An imbalance of certain biochemicals in the brains of overweight people is an inherited condition and is largely responsible for the food obsessions and cravings that drive you to eat too much. It's virtually impossible to control these cravings for any length of time by willpower alone. That's where the use of supplements comes in. The pills restore a proper chemical balance to the brain, which in turn relieves you of cravings and allows you to comfortably reduce the amount of food you eat, especially fat.

Q: **If genetics causes me to be fat, why was I a thin child and teenager?**

A: Most often, genes don't express themselves until later in life. People with highly hereditary diseases,

such as diabetes, high blood pressure, and even
cancer, usually develop them as adults, when a
stressful life event stimulates a genetic dysfunction. The event may be an emotional stressor, pregnancy, change in career or marriage, death of a
loved one, or even a new medication. These things
can trigger the genetic process that leads to an
imbalance in your brain chemistry, which shifts up
the brain thermostat and flips on the hunger
switch, causing uncontrolled weight gain.

Q: What can I do when my weight loss just stops?

A: This can be a difficult problem since it is hard to
know if the brain has reached a new set point or a
temporary plateau. You can try increasing your
supplement dosages as long as you stay within the
safe limits I've talked about earlier. If you've arrived
at a new set point, however, your weight will probably not drop further, because you've reached your
ideal weight—no matter what the insurance charts
say. Your brain determines your particular ideal
body weight. It doesn't care what the average
weight is for your height; it will take you where it
wants you to go, and even using supplements will
not push it further.

Q: Do I have to stay on supplements forever?

A: Most people, but not all, need some kind of maintenance dose. A few are able to maintain weight
loss through diet and exercise (although exercise
won't help you lose weight, it does have a very

small effect on keeping weight off). More often than not, once the pills stop, the brain thermostat starts to move upward, and the lost pounds return. Fortunately, taking supplements just three times a week can very adequately maintain weight loss, especially when combined with very moderate lifestyle changes.

Q: Can you be too thin?

A: Certainly anorexia is too thin and very dangerous. Not eating at all is obviously unhealthy and can lead to serious illness and sudden death. But the fact is that very lean men and women statistically live the longest. A study of 62,000 men and 260,000 women showed that the very thin, with BMIs of only 19 to 22, had the lowest risk of premature death from any cause. This is a very lean weight, but not model thin. Monkeys who are fed a low-calorie diet and are leaner than others often live twice as long than their heavier counterparts. Thin is healthy—but not to the point of starvation.

Q: How much of a problem does obesity really create?

A: Every year, obesity is responsible for more than $70 billion in health care costs and 300,000 deaths in the United States alone. It contributes to heart disease, high blood pressure, stroke, breast and colon cancer, some forms of diabetes, gallbladder disease, and lung disease. Only smoking is more dangerous.

Q: Is childhood overeating a serious risk later in life?

A: Unfortunately, it can be a serious risk. If a child consumes 240 excess calories daily, his or her cancer risk as an adult increases 15 to 20 percent. And the risk rises even higher as the number of daily calories goes up. Overeating can be very difficult to control, since brain chemistry imbalances are driving up the child's appetite and cravings. Once again, this is not a matter of willpower, but we don't want to put children on diets or supplements either. How to deal with this problem in children is obviously highly controversial.

Q: What are realistic weight-loss expectations?

A: Bariatricians consider a weight loss of 10 percent of body weight a success—especially if it can be maintained. This translates into a loss of 25 pounds for a 250-pound woman. Most people would find this result disappointing. In fact, studies show that the average 250-pound woman would only be happy with a 55- to 77-pound weight loss. While this is very understandable, it's not particularly realistic in all cases.

Q: Can stress cause weight gain?

A: Absolutely, even without changing your eating behavior, stress will cause weight gain. It is so powerful that even with supplements, weight will go up. This is due to the tremendous release of stress hormones, one called *cortisol* in particular. Interestingly, this kind or stress response is most common in people who are already overweight. Thin people will often stop eating and lose weight under stress. Again, this represents a difference in brain chemistry and is clearly not a function of willpower or self-control.

Q: Is seasonal depression related to increased food cravings in fall and winter months?

A: You may have seen articles in the popular press about something called "seasonal affective disorder" (SAD), which is a state of depression that begins in autumn, gradually worsens during winter, and disappears with the advent of spring. Research has shown that this depression coincides with a drop in serotonin levels. The theory states that fewer hours of daylight at this time of year trigger a serotonin-sparing response in the brain. That would certainly explain why these people show such marked improvement when they use Prozac, a drug that increases serotonin levels. Many also experience an increase in cravings and food obsessions during the fall and winter. Although we have traditionally blamed seasonal weight gain on holiday meals, it may be that changing balances of brain chemistry increase food cravings as well as depression.

Q: Does taking estrogen pills make weight loss more difficult?

A: Yes. Estrogen promotes fat storage, which really isn't surprising when you think about it. The female hormones your body naturally produces are designed to prepare you for pregnancy and childbirth. This means storing fat, especially in the hips and thighs. Unfortunately, your body doesn't know the difference between an estrogen pill and natural estrogen, so if you're taking this medication, you will probably have more difficulty losing weight.

Q: Why do my food cravings get so intense right before menstruation?

A: Once again, serotonin is the answer. In the premenstrual phase of your cycle, levels drop. Because serotonin is the chemical that keeps you calm, not having enough of it causes you to get irritable and anxious—and to crave sweets and starches.

Q: What about the use of fluid pills or diuretics for weight control?

A: There are absolutely no indications for the use of diuretics in a weight-loss program, and they can dangerously lower your blood pressure and potassium levels. Remember, losing fluid is not the same as losing fat. If you sweat out 8 ounces of perspiration when you exercise, you'll gain it back with your next glass of water. If you're trying to lose weight, diuretics are not an option.

Q: Do you use any behavior modification techniques?

A: Behavior modification for obesity can be broken down into three steps. First, you must identify those factors that lead to overeating, such as particularly tempting foods, emotional stress, social situations, etc. Next, you put obstacles and distractions on the road between temptation and giving in. For example, if you find yourself mesmerized by the dessert buffet at a wedding reception, you might step outside for a walk or drink a very large glass of water or find a partner and dance that polka the band is playing. Finally, you reward yourself for a job well done by giving yourself a little pat on the back whenever you resist a particularly strong temptation.

Behavior modification is great as part of an overall program. By itself, however, it yields disappointing results because it treats symptoms rather than the underlying illness. It does not make food obsessions and cravings go away, and people who suffer the assault of these impulses twenty-four hours a day are likely to give in sooner or later. That means the weight comes back. In my opinion, the problem of brain neurotransmitter levels must be addressed.

Q: Do weight-loss supplements work for everyone?

A: In my experience, weight-loss supplements are effective in about 95 percent of patients. "Effective" means that the average patient will lose 10 percent of her starting body weight in three to six months. In my experience, the patient who does not lose weight on the Hunger Switch program is very rare indeed.

Q: How do I set my goal weight?

A: To be frank, I don't think setting a goal weight is a good idea. It's too easy to set yourself up for failure with unrealistic expectations. Instead, every pound lost should be cause for celebration. Losing 20 pounds will give you significant health benefits and a much improved image of yourself. If you're 100 to 150 pounds overweight, don't even worry about your ideal body weight. Getting there may not be reasonable and probably isn't necessary. If you lose 10 percent of your body weight and keep it off in the long term, you have, in my opinion, accomplished something great.

Having said all this, I realize that many people will insist upon having a way to know when they've lost enough weight. Okay, then, here it is: Listen to your own body. After you have been taking supplements for a while—no one can predict for how long—you will reach a plateau in your weight loss. Nothing you do—not limiting calories, stopping and restarting your supplements, or raising their dosages—will budge the scale. Your body will be telling you that it's at the weight it prefers. Only very extreme, almost obsessive exercising will make any more weight come off. If there is any such thing as a goal or ideal or baseline weight, this is the way in which you will know you have reached it.

Q: Can being overweight lead to arthritis and other painful problems?

A: Unfortunately, yes. We have long suspected that the extra stress and strain inflicted on the joints of overweight people might cause inflammation or arthritis. Recently, a study done by Dr. Allan Gelber, a rheumatologist at Johns Hopkins, confirmed our suspicions. Men who are even moderately overweight are at significantly greater risk for arthritis of the hips and knees. Gelber's study focused on osteoarthritis, which is a painful joint condition that results from the loss of cartilage, a tissue that acts as a shock absorber for the bones. When cartilage wears thin, the joints become warm, swollen, stiff, and painful. The condition afflicts about a third of all people over the age of sixty-five but appears in overweight people far sooner—sometimes as early as twenty years of age.

Q: Should I totally avoid fatty foods?

A: No. In fact, it's not a good idea. You need small amounts of fatty acids to maintain good health. But even if you could avoid them, would you want to? Do you really want to give up all of your favorite foods? You need to indulge yourself now and then to give yourself some pleasure. One of the reasons these natural supplements work so well is that they allow you to eat "junk" food now and then without worry. The difference will be that you won't feel any need to overeat. You'll find you can enjoy a few potato chips or a single scoop of ice cream and be satisfied.

Q: What medications are weight gainers?

A: Many! The biggest offenders are antihistamines, used for allergies; antiseizure drugs; beta-blockers, used for hypertension and migraines; estrogen; and almost all antidepressants, unless they're used in combination with something to balance norepinephrine levels. Furthermore, weight gain can occur very rapidly from the brain chemistry changes induced by these medications. This sets off the entire genetic cascade of events leading to significant weight gain. Unfortunately, drug-induced weight gain is extremely difficult to take off without the help of weight-reducing agents. This particular problem is very frustrating, since the offending medication is often vital for the patient's overall health. I have found that weight-loss agents are the only answer to this dilemma.

Q: **This is confusing because I've heard that Prozac will make you lose weight. Is this true?**

A: Prozac can have that effect for the initial two to three months. After that period, weight gain almost always occurs. But some of the other SSRIs, such as Paxil, are even worse.

Q: **What about blood pressure supplements and weight gain?**

A: Some notorious weight gainers are the diuretics like hydrochlorothiazide, the calcium channel blocker verapamil, and the beta-blockers like propanolol and atanolol. Good alternatives are the ACE inhibitors (of which there are many), which are relatively side effect free, easy to use, and inexpensive.

The beta-blocker Pindolol™ is also a very good choice.

Q: What can I take for allergies?

A: Beware of all antihistamines—even the newer ones. They're weight gainers. For allergy symptoms, try a local steroid nasal spray. Use Sudafed™ for congestion and Tylenol™ for discomfort. There are various eye drops available for itchy eyes—ask your doctor about them. Daily antihistamines are particularly troublesome.

Q: Can I use any antidepressants and not gain weight?

A: Wellbutrin is probably the safest, as far as gaining weight is concerned, but it isn't for everyone. People with seizures can't use it, and it sometimes "wires" people too much. Also, it doesn't raise serotonin levels, so it's not always an ideal antidepressant. Again, if you have any weight problem and you use a serotonin antidepressant, a norepinephrine-balancing substance should be used along with it. You can try ephedra/caffeine, or you can see your family doctor and ask him about taking phentermine.

Appendix

Programs at a Glance

The chart on page 142 offers a quick and easy reference for each profile. Do not mix supplements and medications that do exactly the same thing. For example, do not mix SAM-e and phenylalanine. Also, do not use S-Profile supplements if you are using an SSRI (selective serotonin reuptake inhibitor) for depression.

Natural Supplements

	Ma Huang or Country Mallow (Ephedra)	Green Tea Extract (Caffeine)	Tyrosine	5-HTP (Sublingual)	5-HTP (Supplement)	SAM-e (L-methionine & S-adenosyl)	Phenylalanine
N-PROFILE (*hunger, ADD, insatiability, cravings, exhaustion, depression*)	From 6 mg to 24 mg at 11:00 A.M. and 4:00 P.M.	200 mg twice a day	250–1,000 mg 2 times a day	—	—	—	—
S-PROFILE (*sweet cravings, compulsive eating, food obsession, bingeing, depression, anxiety/panic, phobias*)	From 6 mg to 24 mg at 11:00 A.M. and 4:00 P.M.	200 mg twice a day	—	As needed to curb cravings (with ephedra or phentermine) **OR**	50–100 mg 3 times a day 20 minutes before meals	—	—
D-PROFILE (*depression, addictions, sexual dysfunction, cravings for fatty or salty foods*)	From 6 mg to 24 mg at 11:00 A.M. and 4:00 P.M.	200 mg twice a day	—	As needed to curb cravings (with ephedra or phentermine) **OR**	50–100 mg 3 times a day 20 minutes before meals	1–3 grams a day with a B_6 supplement **OR**	200 mg a day
C-PROFILE (*Supplements alone don't work*)	From 6 mg to 24 mg at 11:00 A.M. and 4:00 P.M.	200 mg twice a day	—	As needed to curb cravings (with ephedra or phentermine) **OR**	50–100 mg 3 times a day 20 minutes before meals	1–3 grams a day with a B_6 supplement **OR**	200 mg a day + Low Carb Diet

Note: For maintenance, take supplements only on Monday, Wednesday, and Friday, or take them every day and cut the dosage in half.

References

Atkinson, R. Report on the NIH workshop on pharmacologic treatment of obesity. *Am J Clin Nutr* 1994; 60:153–56.

Bjorntorp, P. Metabolic implications of body fat distribution. *Diabetes Care* 1991; 14:1132–43.

Bogardus, C. Familial dependence of the metabolic rate. *NEJM* 1986; 315:96–100.

Bray, G. A., and D. S. Gray. Obesity, Part I: Pathogenesis. *West J Med* 1988; 149:429–41.

Bray G. A. Obesity, Part II: Treatment. *West J Med* 1988; 149:555.

Canning, H. Obesity: its possible effects on college admissions. *NEJM* 1966; 275:1172–74.

Clancy, Stephen. *Inter Jour of Sport Nut* 1994; 4:142–53.

DiPasquale, M. G. *Anabolic Research Rev* 2(1):6–10

Douglas, J. G. Drug treatment and obesity. *Pharmacol Ther* 1982; 18:351–73.

Evans, G. W. The effects of chromium picolinate on insulin controlled parameters in humans. *Int Jour Biosocial Med Res* 1989; 11:163–80.

GHB Withdrawal Syndrome Documented. *Annals of Emergency Medicine* (February 2001).

Guy-Grand, B. International trial of long-term dexfenfluramine in obesity. *The Lancet* 1989; 1142–44.

Huang, M. H., R. C. Yang, and S. H. Hu. *Inter Jour of Obesity* 1996; 20(9): 930–36.

Hubert, H. B. The importance of obesity in the development of coronary risk factors and disease. *Ann Rev Pub Health* 1986; 7:493–98.

Jones, Dennis. Essential fatty acids. *Product Monograph* (March 1993).

Le Favi, Robert. *Inter Jour of Sport Nut* 1992; 2:11–122.

Maddox, G. L. Overweight as a social disability with medical implications. *J Med Educ* 1969; 44:214–20.

Mayer, J. Genetic factors in human obesity. *Ann NY Acad Sci* 1965; 131:412–21.

National Institutes of Health Consensus Department Conference. Health implications of obesity. *Ann Intern Med* 1985; 103:977.

Neurosurgical Gamma Knife May Help Treat Obesity. *UniSci Newsletter* http://unisci.com/stories/19994/1029991.htm

Obesity Research Update 2 (March 1977).

Raloff, J. Boning up on calcium shouldn't be sporadic. *Science News* 2000; 157:260.

———. Calcium may become a dieter's best friend. *Science News* 2000; 157:260.

Roe, D. A. Relationship between obesity and associated health factors with unemployment among low-income women. *J Am Med Wom Assoc* 1976; 31:193–94, 198–99, 203–204.

Serotonin and Judgement. *Brain Briefings* (April 1997). http://www.sfn.org/briefings/serotonin.html

Shi, H., and M. B. Zemel. Effects of dietary calcium on adipocyte lipid metabolism and body weight regulation in energy-restricted mice. *FASEB Journal* March 15, 2000; 14:A790.

Staffler, J. R. A study of social stereotype of body image in children. *J Pers Soc Psychol* 1967; 7:101–104.

Stanko, R.T., D. L. Tietze, and J. E. Arch. Body composition, energy utilization, and nitrogen metabolism with a 4-25-MJ/d low-energy diet supplemented with pyruvate. *Amer Jour of Int Nut,* 1992; 56:630–35.

Stunkard, Albert J. The Salmon lecture, "Some Perspectives on Human Obesity; Treatment." *Bull NY Acad Med* 1988; 64:924–40.

UB dental researchers find obesity related to gum disease. *Univ of Buffalo News* 2000.

Univ of Calif Wellness Letter 1997; 13(5):1.

Van Italic, T. B. Health implications of overweight and obesity in the United States. *Ann Intern Med* 1985; 103:983–88.

Weintraub, M. Long-term weight control. *Clin Pharmacol and Ther* 1992; 51:585–646.

Index